Fitness
RUNNING

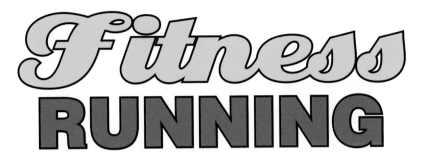

RUNNING

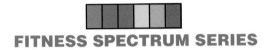

FITNESS SPECTRUM SERIES

Richard L. Brown
Joe Henderson

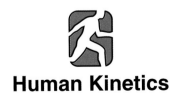

Human Kinetics

Library of Congress Cataloging-in-Publication Data

Brown, Dick., 1937-
   Fitness running / Richard L. Brown, Joe Henderson.
      p.   cm.
   Includes index.
   ISBN 0-87322-451-5
   1. Running. 2. Physical fitness. I. Henderson, Joe, 1943- .
  II. Title.
   GV1061.B77   1994   93-27143
   796.42--dc20   CIP

ISBN: 0-87322-451-5

Copyright © 1994 by Human Kinetics Publishers, Inc.

Developmental Editor: Marni Basic; **Series Consultant:** Brian Sharkey; **Assistant Editor**: Anna Curry; **Copyeditor:** Tom Rice; **Proofreader:** Julia Anderson; **Indexer:** Theresa J. Schaefer; **Photo Editor:** Valerie Hall; **Production Director:** Ernie Noa; **Typesetter:** Ruby Zimmerman; **Text Designer:** Keith Blomberg; **Layout Artist:** Tara Welsch; **Cover Designer:** Jack Davis; **Cover photo:** Wilmer Zehr; **Models:** Jill Bonwell and Joe Seeley (interior), Teri Selin and Paul Selin (cover); **Interior photos:** credits on p. 173; **Interior art:** Keith Neely and Gretchen Walters; **Printer:** Bang Printing

Human Kinetics books are available at special discounts for bulk purchase. Special editions or book excerpts can also be created to specification. For details, contact the Special Sales Manager at Human Kinetics.

Printed in the United States of America   10 9 8 7 6 5 4 3 2

Human Kinetics
P.O. Box 5076, Champaign, IL 61825-5076
1-800-747-4457

Canada: Human Kinetics, Box 24040, Windsor, ON N8Y 4Y9
1-800-465-7301 (in Canada only)

Europe: Human Kinetics, P.O. Box IW14, Leeds LS16 6TR, England
(44) 532 781708

Australia: Human Kinetics, Unit 5, 32 Raglan Avenue,
Edwardstown 5039, South Australia
(08) 371 3755

New Zealand: Human Kinetics, P.O. Box 105-231, Auckland 1
(09) 309 2259

Contents

PART I

PREPARING TO RUN

You already know how to run. It's part of your ancestry and your upbringing.

Humans are a running species, and all children are runners from their first steps. Few of us run right into adulthood, but we all know well the basic technique of putting one foot in front of the other at a faster-than-walking pace.

So the question you want answered in this book isn't, How do I run? but, How can I run *better*? The answers depend on who you are and exactly what "better" means to you.

Let's say you ran high school track, but that was many years and many pounds ago. The longer you've lapsed, the longer and more carefully you must work back into running shape. We'll show you the path to better basic fitness.

Perhaps you already run, but your daily 2 miles through the neighborhood aren't pleasant. You get hurt too often, or you feel physically or mentally flat too much of the time. We'll show you better ways of training without straining.

Maybe you're running trouble-free but want more from your activity. You see ads for a local 5K (3.1-mile) race and wonder, Do I dare enter it? We'll show you how much better running can be when you make it a social event.

You've tried a race and now want to run farther or faster. You aim to improve your PR (personal record) in the 5K, to go for a 10K next time, or to increase your distances all the way up to a marathon. We'll show you how to race better.

In this opening section of the book, we prepare you for your next step forward in running. We lay the groundwork for that progress by addressing and assessing basic requirements for all runners:

- Judging the benefits of running compared to other physical activities
- Choosing proper shoes, clothing, and other equipment to protect you against all weather and surface conditions
- Testing your physical readiness to start running or to adopt a more demanding training program
- Refining your running technique so you can move more smoothly, swiftly, and safely
- Adding warm-up and cool-down periods, as well as supplementing your training menu with flexibility and strength exercises

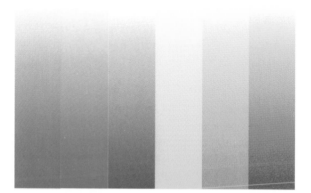

1

Running for Fitness

Running isn't what it used to be. It's bigger and better, offering you more than ever before.

Consider the case of Richard Benyo, now a prominent running writer. He has seen both sides of running, the before and the after. Benyo first ran as a high school and college track and cross-country athlete, which was about the only reason anyone ran in the 1960s. He then retired from the sport, as runners were expected to do back then. Benyo remained inactive until his weight crept up to an intolerable figure. He then returned to running and found it a much different sport than the one he'd left a decade earlier. People were now running for exercise. They were running road races. The middle-aged and elderly were running. Women were running.

Benyo faced a smorgasbord of choices, and he sampled them all: exercise running, racing for fun, serious racing at distances up to the 26-mile marathon, and adventure running at distances beyond 100 miles.

He found a career in running, first as an editor at *Runner's World* magazine and later as the author of several running books. Benyo had found a sport that could last him a lifetime. So did hundreds of thousands of runners. And so can you.

Who Runs What?

Various national polls taken in the early 1990s pegged the total number of U.S. runners at more than 20 million. How true this figure is depends on how strictly you define the word *runner*.

The National Sporting Goods Association (NSGA) asked how often individuals ran, setting as its minimum standard 5 or more days of running in the past year. Some 21.8 million Americans ran at least that often in 1991, according to the NSGA survey.

Even more exciting than the overall growth of running has been the spread of running to groups that once ignored the activity. As recently as the 1960s, it was confined largely to males in their teens to early 20s who ran races. Running has since opened up to women, and now it holds great appeal to older age groups.

Men still outnumbered women in the NSGA survey, but only 59% to 41%. Women have narrowed that gap with each new poll. The age group

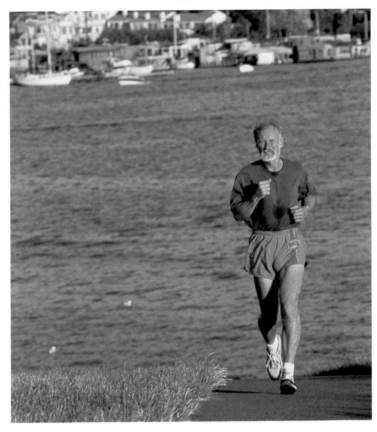

Age is just a number to a runner.

with the most runners of both sexes was 35 to 54. The average age of runners has increased in each poll.

Most of the millions of runners counted in the NSGA poll probably ran too little to meet minimum fitness needs, which requires running at least 3 days a week. A survey taken by American Sports Data in early 1992 identified the number of runners who trained 150 or more days a year (or slightly less than three times weekly). Some 5.4 million qualified.

The easiest headcount to take is runners entering U.S. road races. They tend to be the best trained, and their numbers are increasing. The country's largest running events are growing the fastest, according to the national Road Running Information Center. Total entrants in the 100 biggest races grew by 69% (to 807,000) in the 1982-91 decade.

Race participation in events of all sizes continues to grow at the rate of about 5% a year. It now totals more than 1.5 million racers, and you're welcome to join them if you wish. These races accept runners from every level of ability and every degree of ambition.

Why Run?

Running has less going for it than most other physical activity programs, and the word *less* is its primary attraction. It requires less learning time, less training time, less equipment, and less organization than almost any other fitness routine we could name.

Consider the strengths of running:

- **Simplicity**. There is little need to learn skills, hire an instructor, join a club, find a field or court or companion, or do anything but lace up your running shoes and head out the door.
- **Efficiency**. Few other activities match running's physical benefits per minute of activity. You can accomplish maximum work in minimum time. All but the most advanced training programs require no more than 1 or 2 hours a week to complete.
- **Economy**. Running is a relatively cheap activity. The one essential purchase is a good pair of shoes. There are many other ways to spend your money on running, but most of these deal with optional equipment or trips to races.
- **Objectivity**. Running is one of the most easily measured activities. You measure yourself primarily against the objective standards of time and distance, not against an opponent.
- **Democracy**. Everyone is welcome. You can share the same race starting line with the best runners in the world. You can put in as much effort and feel what they feel during and after the race.
- **Freedom**. It can be either a social or a solitary activity. The choice is yours, and it can vary from day to day.

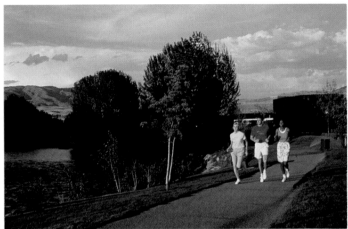

Running with others is an opportunity to squeeze fitness and friendship into one time slot.

As with any strenuous physical activity, running also involves trade-offs. Along with the many pluses just named, you need to be aware of some minuses and how to overcome them.

The downside of running centers on two areas:

- **Injuries**. The injury risk is real. One runner in every two experiences some form of injury in any year. But because these injuries usually result from training mistakes, they rarely are severe or permanent.
- **Imbalances**. Running is an incomplete exercise. It develops a specialized set of muscles at the expense of others. It works best in combination with other supplementary strength and flexibility exercises. (See chapter 5 for recommended exercises.)

The F-I-T Formula

All worthwhile aerobic training programs—whether for casual exercise running or for serious competitive training—address three basic questions: how long? how hard? how often?

The basic fitness formula can be expressed as the acronym *FIT*. It stands for *frequency* (how often you train), *intensity* (how hard you train), and *time* (how long you train).

You must train often enough, hard enough, and long enough to stimulate the improvements you're seeking. And yet you must balance the work with recovery, or you'll risk exhaustion and injury that halt your progress. All training is a balancing act between "enough" and "too much."

Training needs also are personal, varying according to the individual runner's ability and ambition.

Keeping these facts in mind, we offer training plans in Part III that can be tailored to your own fitness and goals. These training programs target three levels of running, each having its own FIT guidelines:

- **Beginning/Easy running** treats running primarily as a way to meet the minimum standards of aerobic fitness. The beginning programs are for those who have little interest in pushing the limits of distance or speed. They include 3 to 4 days of running per week, with an average running time of 20 to 35 minutes, and 0 or 1 hard runs per week.

- **Frequent/Moderate running** combines the exercise with some low-key pushing of limits. These programs are geared toward runners who enjoy occasionally running farther or faster than they need to do for basic fitness. The frequent running programs include 3 to 5 days of running per week, with an average running time of 20 to 45 minutes, and 1 hard run per week.

- **Competitive/Intense running** emphasizes improving one's performances. The competitive programs are for those who train harder than the other types of runners and often put that training to test in races. These programs include 4 to 6 days of running per week, with an average running time of 20 minutes to 1 hour, and 1 or 2 hard runs per week.

Benefits of Running

We've compiled a scorecard on running, rating its benefits in five aspects of physical fitness. Those fitness factors are as follows (see Figure 1.1 for comparisons of running with other popular fitness activities):

- **Body composition**. Running receives a high mark for benefits in body composition. Of the six activities we compare, none has a more dramatic effect in trimming away unwanted fat than running. It is a calorie burner par excellence.

   Running further benefits body composition in these ways: Increased calcium deposits mean stronger bones, and increased blood supply means stronger ligaments and tendons in the lower body. (The upper body receives only partial benefits in these respects.)

- **Cardiovascular fitness**. Running again receives highest marks for improving the efficiency of your circulatory system. This allows you to exercise longer and exhibit greater effort without exhausting yourself.

   Increased heart volume and contractile force mean more blood is pumped per beat. Increased heart vascularization means more blood

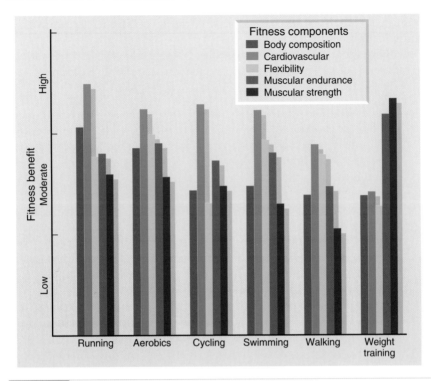

Figure 1.1   How running compares to other fitness activities.

is supplied to the heart muscle. Increased blood volume and a higher red-blood-cell count mean more oxygen-carrying capacity.

- **Flexibility**. Running doesn't give your muscles much of a stretch. In fact, it may decrease overall flexibility enough to increase the risk of injury.

    Running trails several other activities (notably swimming and aerobic dance) in this regard. We recommend that you supplement your workouts with flexibility exercises. (You'll find suggested stretching exercises in chapter 5.)

- **Muscle endurance**. Runners develop the ability to withstand long periods of work. But weight trainers display much more muscle endurance, so we advise you to add weight training to your routine.

    Running increases the muscles' energy-producing ability, particularly in the lower body. (The upper body benefits less in this way.) Over time, increased energy production will translate into a greater capacity to perform prolonged work.

- **Muscle strength**. Running increases muscle protein, which leads to stronger muscles. This trait translates into runners' explosive power, or the ability to accelerate quickly to high speed.

  Running itself develops only fair muscle strength, and this primarily in the lower body. Again, you might want to adopt some weight work. Figure 1.2 shows how running affects the muscles.

Running offers an attractive physical fitness package. None of the activities we compare it with score better across the board. Now that we've shown you this sport's promise, let's get you better equipped for running itself.

ASSESSING YOUR PHYSICAL READINESS

Running is a strenuous physical activity. Seven questions from the Physical Activity Readiness Questionnaire (PAR-Q) will help you assess your readiness to start running. (See chapter 3 for a further assessment of your health and fitness levels.)

PAR-Q & YOU

		YES	NO
1.	Has your doctor ever said that you have a heart condition *and* that you should only do physical activity recommended by a doctor?	___	___
2.	Do you feel pain in your chest when you do physical activity?	___	___
3.	In the past month, have you had chest pain when you were not doing physical activity?	___	___
4.	Do you lose your balance because of dizziness or do you ever lose consciousness?	___	___
5.	Do you have a bone or joint problem that could be made worse by a change in your physical activity?	___	___
6.	Is your doctor currently prescribing drugs (for example, water pills) for your blood pressure or heart condition?	___	___
7.	Do you know of *any other reason* why you should not do physical activity?	___	___

If you answer yes to any question, go no further until you receive a doctor's clearance. If you answer no to every question, you can be reasonably sure it's safe to increase your physical activity.

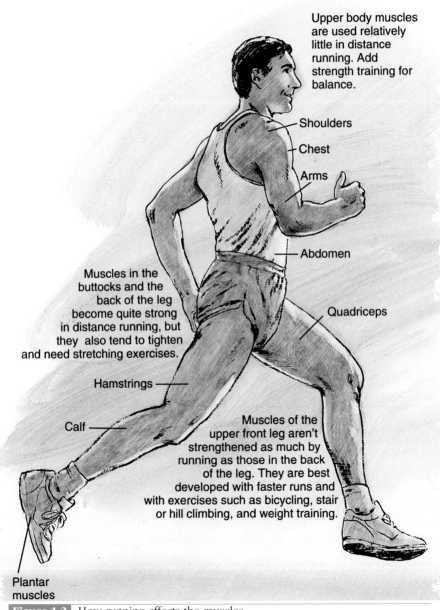

Upper body muscles are used relatively little in distance running. Add strength training for balance.

Shoulders

Chest

Arms

Abdomen

Muscles in the buttocks and the back of the leg become quite strong in distance running, but they also tend to tighten and need stretching exercises.

Quadriceps

Hamstrings

Calf

Muscles of the upper front leg aren't strengthened as much by running as those in the back of the leg. They are best developed with faster runs and with exercises such as bicycling, stair or hill climbing, and weight training.

Plantar muscles

Figure 1.2 How running affects the muscles.

2

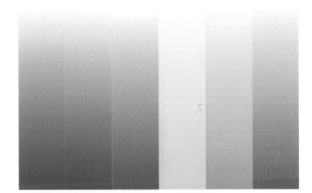

Getting Equipped

Part of running's beauty lies in its simplicity. What could be more basic than lacing up a good pair of running shoes, slipping into the right clothing for the conditions, and heading out your front door for a run?

Okay, maybe outfitting yourself for walking is even simpler. But your essential equipment purchases for running are few and relatively inexpensive compared to most other sports.

We'll advise you in this chapter on buying shoes, clothing, and accessories. We'll also remind you that another vital raw material of running, a place to practice this activity, is as free and unlimited as the world outside your door.

The Well-Dressed Runner

You can, if so inclined, dress colorfully and stylishly for running. Or you can wear your old, baggy gray sweats.

You can spend hundreds of dollars on the highest tech shoes and the latest miracle fibers that both look great and feel great. Or you can make minimal, but still quite functional, purchases at a discount or secondhand store.

Which way you dress up—or down—to run depends on your budget and fashion sense. We deal here only with the few essentials.

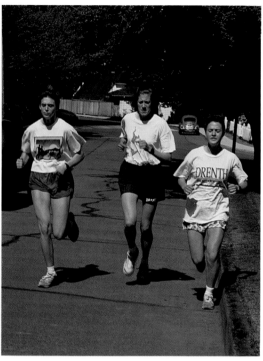

A pair of good running shoes, an old T-shirt and shorts, and you're ready to run.

The list starts with shoes, and maybe it could end with them. Even if you don't already run, your wardrobe probably holds all the clothes you need to start running.

Almost any light, nonrestrictive clothing will work early on. But you can't run well in just any old shoes.

Shoes

You need shoes made specifically for running because runners strike the ground with a force three or more times their body weight; the ground they strike is usually paved and unyielding, and running shoes are specially designed to absorb this shock.

High-quality running shoes feature several layers of cushioning underneath the entire foot, slight elevation of the heel, flexibility of the forefoot, and protection against excessive side-to-side motion. All of this comes in a relatively lightweight package.

Good shoes cost $40 to $100. You can find look-alikes for less than $40, but they're rarely bargains because they lack essential design features or durability. You also can pay more than $100, but you're probably paying for an overdesigned shoe that won't noticeably help your running.

You're wise to stick with the established running shoe makers. *Runner's World* magazine deems these companies worthy of inclusion in its annual shoe surveys: Adidas, Asics, Avia, Brooks, Diadora, Etonic, Mizuno, New Balance, Nike, Reebok, Saucony, and Turntec.

For specific shoes recommendations, check the reports in *Runner's World* and *Running Times*. Then go to a running specialty store, whose staff is trained to help you make the right selection and ensure proper fit. You aren't home-free once you've bought the right shoes. You still need to deal with several aspects of shoe wear and care to enjoy trouble-free running:

- **Shoe break-in**. Even well-made running shoes require a breaking-in period. You should be able to put on a new pair and run without blistering, but any new shoes will cause you to hit the ground differently than you did in the old pair. You may develop soreness in your feet and legs while adapting to this change, so use the new shoes only for your easier runs until you've adapted fully.
- **Shoe care**. Well-used running shoes get dirty and smelly. But because they're made mostly of synthetic materials, they can be washed. Hose them off frequently or throw them in the washer, but let them dry in the sun instead of the dryer to prevent damage. You may want to buy two pairs of shoes so you'll have a dry pair each day.
- **Shoe wear**. Running shoes wear out two ways. The soles and heels grind down, of course, but the cushioning materials also fatigue and compress. You can repair the outer surfaces, but the shoe won't be as good as new if compression has changed the original shape and thickness of the sole. Most running shoes need to be replaced after 500 to 1000 miles of wear.
- **Shoe inserts**. You can make a good shoe better by inserting protective devices. These include insoles to replace those provided by the shoe manufacturer, upgraded arch supports, heel cushions, and custom-made shoe inserts called *orthotics*. The first three products are sold in sports stores, and the orthotics are prescribed by a doctor. Use these devices only if you are troubled by injuries.

Clothing

Whether you outfit yourself from a specialty store or from items you already own, include the following in your running wardrobe:

- Underwear that supports without binding
- Socks that don't slip down and bunch up in your shoes to cause blisters

- Shorts that allow freedom of movement and don't irritate your inner thighs
- A variety of shirts—turtleneck, long-sleeved, short-sleeved, and sleeveless—in a variety of fabrics and weights
- Gloves or mittens to warm the part of you that gets cold the quickest
- Several types of headwear—stocking cap for cold; cap with a facemask for extreme cold; baseball-style cap with visor to protect against rain, sun, or blinding headlights
- Tights that protect against the cold, and don't get baggy and heavy in the rain
- Sweats, windbreakers, or weatherproof suits—both jacket and pants—to keep you cozy in the worst conditions

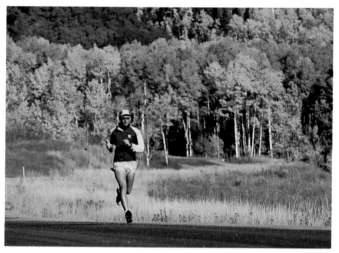

The beauty of running—color-coordinated outfits are optional.

Other Equipment

Your smallest piece of equipment is one of the most useful tools—a digital watch. Its stopwatch feature will give you instant, accurate feedback on your runs. A higher tech (and therefore more expensive) feedback device is the heart-rate monitor. It registers the level of effort that you're putting into a workout.

Sunglasses have become a standard piece of equipment for many runners. The shades reduce tension-causing glare and perhaps prevent eye damage in bright sunlight.

If you require entertainment while running, take along a stereo headset if you plan to run on a track or a running trail. But if you run on the street, be warned that tuning in those sounds and tuning out traffic noises can be hazardous to your health.

Adding Up the Costs

How much it will cost to outfit yourself for running depends on how frugally or royally you wish to be outfitted. First, we list the rock-bottom costs, then the high-end purchases.

Low-Budget Dressing

Limit your shopping list to a single item: shoes. Choose shoes made specifically for running from one of the major manufacturers listed in this chapter. Look for bargains among discontinued models and shoes discounted because of cosmetic defects. You should be able to find a pair for $50 or slightly less.

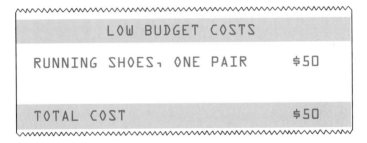

```
LOW BUDGET COSTS

RUNNING SHOES, ONE PAIR        $50


TOTAL COST                     $50
```

Otherwise, dress in clothing that you already own. Use the same wristwatch you now wear, provided it gives accurate readings while running.

High-Budget Dressing

Outfit yourself completely. Splurge on a waterproof, windproof suit and two pairs of high-quality shoes for different types of running (say, training and racing). Buy a runner's wristwatch that tells you everything except what to eat for breakfast.

The prices that follow aren't the highest you can go. You can duplicate other items besides shoes, and add accessories such as a headset, sunglasses, or a heart-rate monitor. We're assuming that you already own suitable hats, gloves, socks, underwear, and T-shirts.

HIGH BUDGET COSTS	
WEATHERPROOF SUIT	$200
RUNNING SHOES, TWO PAIRS	150
RUNNER'S WATCH	45
FULL-LENGTH TIGHTS	40
KNEE-LENGTH TIGHTS	30
LINED SHORTS	20
HOT-WEATHER MESH SINGLET	15
TOTAL COST	$500

Creating a Positive Climate

The weather during running isn't what it appears to be as you prepare to run. Don't believe what you see as you look out the window. Don't believe what the thermometer says.

Winter days won't be as cold as they seem when you start to run. Summer days won't be as perfect as they feel at first. That's because a 20° rule works either for or against a runner. The apparent Fahrenheit temperature will climb by that amount as you hit your stride. (In Celsius, it's about 10°.)

For example, a chilly 40 °F (5 °C) morning will become a pleasant 60 (15 °C). A balmy 75° (24 °C) afternoon will become an unpleasant 95 (34 °C). Your body has a good furnace but a bad air conditioner. It warms up nicely in cold weather but cools down poorly on hot days.

Plan your runs with the 20 °F (10 °C) rule in mind. Dress for the temperature in midrun, not how you feel at the starting line. Dress in layers that can be stripped away as you warm up (jacket, long-sleeved shirt, T-shirt, pants, tights, cap, and gloves).

Run in the cooler hours of a summer day. Save your hardest runs for the coolest days (perhaps those with rain, wind, and clouds). In winter, reverse that pattern. Run during the warmer hours, and run hardest on the warmest days (when the sun is out, the wind is calm, and the roads are clear of snow).

Don't let summer heat or winter cold keep you indoors. A well-dressed runner can train safely in any season. But you still must consider the potential risks that lurk at either extreme of temperature. Hot days carry the risk of heat exhaustion, and cold days the risk of frostbite.

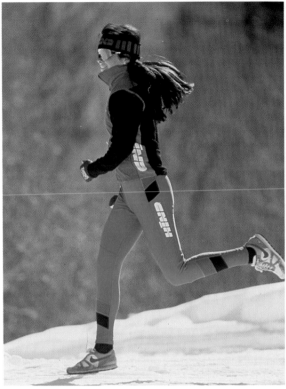

The winter landscape is not off-limits if you're dressed appropriately.

Again, the thermometer may not tell the whole truth. High humidity makes hot days feel hotter than the actual temperature, and high wind makes cold days feel colder. Plan your running and your wardrobe according to the heat-humidity readings in Table 2.1 and wind-chill readings in Table 2.2.

Individuals differ, of course, in their reactions to extreme heat and cold. You also adapt somewhat as you train in them and how you dress for them.

Generally speaking, however, we can rate these conditions by how they affect your running. We've taken National Weather Service readings for heat-humidity and wind-chill, and given them letter grades:

A = good day; B = fair day; C = marginal day; D = poor day; F = unsafe day.

Heat-Humidity Readings

In Table 2.1, find the temperature down the left side of the scale and the humidity level along the top. Go to the point where these two figures meet

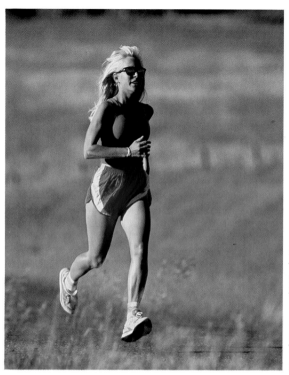

David Epperson/F-Stock, Inc.

Plan what to wear and how hard to run in hot weather according to the temperature and humidity.

Table 2.1
Hot-Weather Ratings

Temp.	Humidity								
	20%	30%	40%	50%	60%	70%	80%	90%	100%
75 °F (24 °C)	A	A	A	A	A	A	A	B	B
80 °F (26 °C)	A	A	A	B	B	C	C	D	D
85 °F (29 °C)	B	B	C	C	D	D	D	F	F
90 °F (32 °C)	C	C	D	D	D	F	F	F	F
95 °F (35 °C)	D	D	F	F	F	F	F	F	F

for the day's grade. Temperatures below 75 °F (24 °C) rate *A*'s and those above 95° (35 °C) are *F*'s at most humidity levels.

Wind-Chill Readings

In Table 2.2, find the wind speed down the left side of the scale and the temperature across the top. Go to the point where these two readings meet for the day's grade. Temperatures above 35 °F (2 °C) rate *A*'s and those below −10° (−23 °C) are *F*'s at most wind speeds.

Table 2.2
Cold-Weather Ratings

				Temperature						
Wind reading	35 °F (1 °C)	30 °F (-1 °C)	25 °F (-3 °C)	20 °F (-6 °C)	15 °F (-8 °C)	10 °F (-10 °C)	5 °F (-12 °C)	0 °F (-15 °C)	-5 °F (-17 °C)	-10 °F (-19 °C)
Calm	A	A	A	B	B	B	B	C	C	C
10 mph	A	B	B	B	C	C	C	D	D	D
20 mph	B	B	C	C	C	D	D	D	F	F
30 mph	C	C	C	D	D	D	F	F	F	F
40 mph	C	C	D	D	D	F	F	F	F	F

Where to Run?

Special tracks or trails are nice bonuses, but you don't require them. Anywhere you could freely and safely walk can become a running course.

A legendary track and field coach, Bill Bowerman, says, "Running country is everywhere. Run right out the door, and you're in business. Run on a city street, on a country road, in a schoolyard, at the beach, or in a vacant lot. Run down a bicycle path, around a golf course, through a park, in your backyard, in a supermarket parking lot. Anywhere."

You can run anywhere, anytime, and in almost any weather conditions. But you must equip yourself according to the clothing guidelines given in this chapter if the running is to be safe, productive, and enjoyable.

Concern over conditions isn't limited to the weather. You must also remain ever watchful of traffic. Most runners train in the streets, sidewalks, and roads, which are accessible in all weather and at all times, day and night. But they also put you in direct competition with vehicles, the single biggest threat to a runner's safety. For your protection, follow these rules of the road:

1. Choose roadways with sidewalks or wide shoulders as your safety zone, running on the left side to face oncoming traffic.
2. Always yield the right of way, assuming that the road belongs to the cars (as well as trucks, motorcycles, and even bicycles), if only because of their size and speed.
3. Never provoke the drivers of these deadly weapons by invading their lane, dashing across in front of them, or berating them in cases of close calls.
4. Do the drivers' thinking for them, anticipating their moves and making eye contact with them at risky crossings.
5. Stay alert, keeping your head up and eyes on the road, and fighting the tendency to daydream the miles away when road conditions would make daydreaming risky.
6. To be seen, wear brightly colored clothing in the daytime and reflective items at night.
7. Hear what's coming, leaving your cassette tape player or earphone radio at home where it won't drown out warnings of danger.

Now you're dressed to run and armed with running's safety rules. You're set to test your readiness for the better runs that lie ahead.

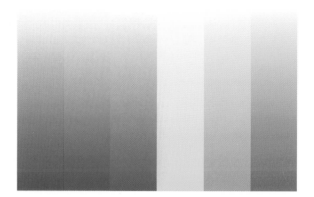

3

Checking Your Running Fitness Level

Your final task before launching into the running program that we prescribe is to determine exactly where your starting point is. In other words, just how healthy and fit are you? This question applies as much to experienced runners as to beginners.

The terms "health" and "fitness" aren't synonymous. Health is merely the absence of disease or injury. Fitness is the ability to perform a specific physical task. You can be healthy in the sense of being illness-free and uninjured, but still unprepared for the performance demands of running. Or you can be fit from recent aerobic training, but unhealthy in the medical sense.

Determine your current levels of health and fitness by taking the two entrance exams in this chapter. Let the results tell you where to begin. Be honest with yourself here. If you ignore key items in your medical history or overestimate your capabilities, the running will make you face the painful truth. To minimize pain and maximize improvement, you must start on the line that is right for you.

Test Your Health/Fitness

We conducted a basic health screening in chapter 1. It asked about high-risk conditions and sent you to a physician if any red flags appeared in your medical records. Here, we offer a self-test that is more specific to running. It checks both your health history and your fitness habits.

Choose the number that best describes you in each of these 10 areas, then add up your score. The results tell whether your starting-line condition is high, average, or low.

ASSESSING YOUR RUNNING FITNESS

Cardiovascular Health

Which of these statements best describes your cardiovascular condition? This is a critical safety check before you enter any vigorous activity. (*Warning:* If you have a history of cardiovascular disease, start the running programs in this book only after receiving clearance from your doctor—and then only with close supervision by a fitness instructor.)

No history of heart or circulatory problems	_____	(3)
Past ailments have been treated successfully	_____	(2)
Such problems exist but no treatment required	_____	(1)
Under medical care for cardiovascular illness	_____	(0)

Injuries

Which of these statements best describes your current injuries? This is a test of your musculoskeletal readiness to start a running program. (*Warning:* If your injury is temporary, wait until it is cured before starting the program. If it is chronic, adjust the program to fit your limitations.)

No current injury problems	_____	(3)
Some pain in activity but not limited by it	_____	(2)
Level of activity is limited by the injury	_____	(1)
Unable to do much strenuous training	_____	(0)

(*continued*)

ASSESSING YOUR RUNNING FITNESS (*continued*)

Illnesses

Which of these statements best describes your current illnesses?
Certain temporary or chronic conditions will delay or disrupt your
running program. (See warning under "Injuries.")

No current illness problems _____ (3)

Some problem in activity but not limited by it _____ (2)

Level of activity is limited by the illness _____ (1)

Unable to do much strenuous training _____ (0)

Age

Which of these age groups describes you? In general, the younger
you are, the less time you have spent slipping out of shape.

Age 19 and younger _____ (3)

Ages 20 to 29 _____ (2)

Ages 30 to 39 _____ (1)

Ages 40 and older _____ (0)

Weight

Which of these figures describes how close you are to your own
definition of "ideal weight"? Excess fat is a major mark of unfitness,
but it's also possible to be significantly underweight.

Within 5 pounds of ideal weight _____ (3)

6 to 10 pounds above or below the ideal _____ (2)

11 to 19 pounds above or below ideal weight _____ (1)

20 or more pounds above or below the ideal _____ (0)

Resting Pulse Rate

Which of these figures describes your current pulse rate on waking
up but before getting out of bed? A well-trained heart beats slower
and more efficiently than one that's unfit.

Below 60 beats per minute _____ (3)

60 to 69 beats per minute _____ (2)

70 to 79 beats per minute _____ (1)

80 or more beats per minute _____ (0)

(continued)

Smoking

Which of these statements best describes your smoking history and current habit (if any)? Smoking is the number one enemy of health and fitness.

Never a smoker _____ (3)

Once a smoker but quit _____ (2)

An occasional, light smoker now _____ (1)

A regular, heavy smoker now _____ (0)

Most Recent Run

Which of these statements best describes your running within the last month? The best single measure of how well you will run in the near future is what you ran in the recent past.

Ran nonstop for more than 2 miles _____ (3)

Ran nonstop for 1 to 2 miles _____ (2)

Ran nonstop for less than 1 mile _____ (1)

No recent run of any distance _____ (0)

Running Background

Which of these statements best describes your running history? Running fitness isn't long-lasting, but the fact that you once ran is a good sign that you can do it again.

Trained for running within the past year _____ (3)

Trained for running 1 to 2 years ago _____ (2)

Trained for running more than 2 years ago _____ (1)

Never trained formally for running _____ (0)

(*continued*)

ASSESSING YOUR RUNNING FITNESS (*continued*)

> ### Related Activities
>
> Which of these statements best describes your participation in other exercises that are similar to running in their aerobic benefit? The closer they relate to running (as do bicycling, swimming, cross-country skiing, and fast walking, for example), the better the carryover effect will be.
>
> Regularly practice similar aerobic activities   _____ (3)
>
> Regularly practice less vigorous aerobics   _____ (2)
>
> Regularly practice nonaerobic sports   _____ (1)
>
> Not regularly active in any physical activity   _____ (0)
>
> **TOTAL SCORE**   _____

If you scored 20 points or more, you rate high in health and fitness for a beginning runner. You probably can handle continuous runs of at least 2 to 3 miles or 20 to 30 minutes.

At 10 to 19 points, your score is average. You may need to take some walking breaks to complete runs of 2 to 3 miles or 20 to 30 minutes.

A score of less than 10 is low. You may need to start with walking only, increasing the sessions to a half-hour before adding any running.

Test Your Running Fitness

Now comes your final exam, so to speak. This is the most telling of the tests, because up to now you've only surveyed your health and fitness with pen and paper. Now you check it where it counts—on the run.

Dr. Kenneth Cooper, the leading authority in aerobic fitness, recommends a 12-minute run (or run-walk mix). See how much distance you can cover in this time period.

The results of this test match up well with those obtained from sophisticated laboratory findings. The key result here is your ability to take in and process the oxygen that fuels your running.

Exercise scientists call this reading *maximal oxygen uptake* and abbreviate it as $\dot{V}O_2max$. The volume (V) of oxygen (O_2) consumed by a person is expressed in milliliters per kilogram of body weight per minute of activity (ml/kg/min).

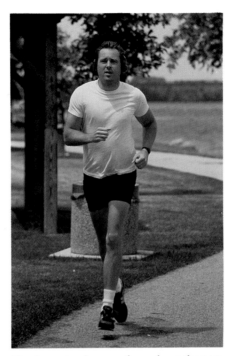

Aim for a steady pace throughout the test.

Generally speaking, the more efficiently you transport and use oxygen, the faster you can run. An inactive adult has a $\dot{V}O_2$max of about 31 ml/kg/min, which enables that person to run a mile in about 9:00. An excellent runner may have a $\dot{V}O_2$max of about 75, which allows that person to run a mile in about 4:10.

If both of these people weigh 70 kilograms (154 pounds), the inactive one will use 19,530 milliliters of oxygen during the mile run. The superfit runner will use 22,052 milliliters.

Looking at these amounts another way, a soft drink can contains 355 milliliters. The sedentary person used 55 cans of oxygen in the mile, while the skilled runner used 62 in less than half the time.

Many authorities use $\dot{V}O_2$max as a benchmark of fitness, as we do in this book. Table 3.1 equates the distance covered in Cooper's 12-minute test with $\dot{V}O_2$max.

12-MINUTE TEST

1. Use a local track or a flat stretch of accurately measured road. (The standard running track is 440 yards or 400 meters. Four laps equal one mile or 1.6 kilometers.)
2. Start at a pace you can maintain throughout the 12 minutes.
3. Increase the pace slightly in the last 1 or 2 minutes.
4. Aim to feel tired but exhilarated at the finish, not exhausted.
5. Look forward to repeating this test in the future with excitement, not with dread.

The farther you run in 12 minutes, the greater your oxygen uptake reading. The less distance you cover within that time limit, the lower your reading.

The results place you into one of four running fitness categories:

- **Superior**, with 2.4 miles or more ($\dot{V}O_2$max of 65 or more)
- **High**, with 1.9 to 2.3 miles ($\dot{V}O_2$max of 50 to 64)
- **Average**, with 1.4 to 1.8 miles ($\dot{V}O_2$max of 35 to 49)
- **Low**, with less than 1.4 miles ($\dot{V}O_2$max below 35)

Grade yourself by the standards in Table 3.1 If your score is low, don't let it discourage you for two reasons:

First, this test score is merely a starting point for your progress. The lower it is, the more room you have for improvement in later tests.

Second, this result gives you a realistic basis for selecting training programs in this book. They must be based on your current ability.

However you train, you must run efficiently. The next chapter instructs you on proper running form.

		Table 3.1	
		Self-Test of Running Fitness	
Laps	**Miles (mile pace)**	**Kilometers (K pace)**	**$\dot{V}O_2$max**
		Low fitness	
4	1.00 (12:00)	1.6 (7:30)	23.7
4-1/4	1.06 (11:19)	1.7 (7:04)	25.4
4-1/2	1.13 (10:37)	1.8 (6:40)	27.2
4-3/4	1.19 (10:05)	1.9 (6:19)	29.1
5	1.25 (9:36)	2.0 (6:00)	30.9
5-1/4	1.31 (9:07)	2.1 (5:43)	32.7
5-1/2	1.38 (8:42)	2.2 (5:27)	34.6
		Average fitness	
5-3/4	1.44 (8:20)	2.3 (5:13)	36.5
6	1.50 (8:00)	2.4 (5:00)	38.4
6-1/4	1.56 (7:42)	2.5 (4:48)	40.3
6-1/2	1.63 (7:22)	2.6 (4:37)	42.2
6-3/4	1.69 (7:06)	2.7 (4:27)	44.2
7	1.75 (6:51)	2.8 (4:17)	46.1
7-1/4	1.81 (6:38)	2.9 (4:08)	48.1
		High fitness	
7-1/2	1.88 (6:23)	3.0 (4:00)	50.1
7-3/4	1.94 (6:11)	3.1 (3:52)	52.1
8	2.00 (6:00)	3.2 (3:45)	54.1
8-1/4	2.06 (5:50)	3.3 (3:38)	56.1
8-1/2	2.13 (5:38)	3.4 (3:31)	58.1
8-3/4	2.19 (5:29)	3.5 (3:25)	60.2
9	2.25 (5:20)	3.6 (3:20)	62.2
9-1/4	2.31 (5:12)	3.7 (3:15)	64.3
		Superior fitness	
9-1/2	2.38 (5:03)	3.8 (3:10)	66.4
9-3/4	2.44 (4:55)	3.9 (3:05)	68.1
10	2.50 (4:48)	4.0 (3:00)	70.6
10-1/4	2.56 (4:41)	4.1 (2:55)	72.7
10-1/2	2.63 (4:34)	4.2 (2:50)	74.6

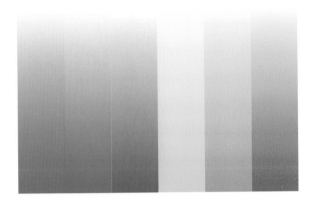

Running the Right Way

Running is as easy as putting one foot in front of the other, you might think. As long as you remember to alternate feet, you can't run into too much trouble, right? Not quite. Running might be this simple if you were blessed with picture-perfect form, but very few of us are. And it might not matter if your technique were ragged if you only ran to catch a bus, but you have bigger plans.

Small mistakes in the way you move can penalize you greatly as your distances grow longer and your speed grows faster. To avoid wasting energy and time, you must pay attention to the details of your running form.

Correct running form covers a wide range of personal differences, but four general rules apply to everyone:

1. **The form must fit the individual. A five-foot-two runner, for instance, can't use the same stride length as someone a foot taller.**
2. **The form must fit the pace. The faster you go, the more you run up on your toes. The slower you run, the more flat-footed you become.**

3. **The form must be mechanically efficient. Humans are upright animals and run best that way—with a straight back.**
4. **The form must be relaxed. Running with tension is like driving a car with its brakes on, causing you to work harder while going slower.**

How do you run? This isn't a question of how far, how fast, or how often. How do you move? You probably haven't thought much about it, and most of the time that's the way to treat this basically automatic action. Running is like breathing. It usually goes along just fine without you thinking about it.

Ken Doherty, a longtime coach and noted writer on running techniques, advises, "Do what comes naturally, as long as 'naturally' is mechanically sound. If it isn't, do what is mechanically sound until it comes naturally."

In this chapter, we look into the mechanics of sound running—from feet to head.

Feet First

Runners fall into two general categories: those who run *on* the ground and try to pound it flat, and those who run *over* the ground, using the earth as a springboard for staying airborne. Let the springboard serve as your model.

Some runners will never sneak up behind you. Without looking over your shoulder, you can hear them coming—Clomp! Clomp! Clomp! You can almost feel their impact. The noise indicates two related problems: overstriding (reaching out too far with the feet) and landing with the knees locked.

Strive for silence in your running. This begins with a knee that is slightly flexed so that it can bend on impact. The foot then lands more directly under the body and at midfoot rather than heel-first. As the ankle unlocks, you rock quickly back onto the heel, then forward again for lift-off.

To put more spring into your run, check the foot, ankle, and knee.

- **Foot.** Make full use of it, from heel to midfoot to toes, as you roll through the running motion. Give a little push with the big toe as you leave the ground.
- **Ankle.** Flex it. Use it to get more bounce. The more rigid the ankle is, the more jarring the contact with the ground will be.
- **Knee.** Lift it. The lift of the knee controls the ball of the foot. If the knee rides low and rigid, your foot will barely clear the ground. Pick up the knee and bend it.

Keep the word "prance" in mind as you perfect your foot-leg action. Run as if you're proud of yourself—quietly proud.

Fully Armed

You see both types. One runs like a boxer, trying to protect the face. The arms ride high and tight, the fists stop just short of the chin, and the shoulders are tense.

The other runner dangles the arms at the sides with fingers pointed at the ground, as if these appendages serve no useful purpose. In neither case do these runners' arms and hands do much good.

In fact, the upper body plays important roles in two-legged locomotion. It counterbalances the action of the legs and provides driving force.

- **Arms**. Your arms swing in rhythm with the legs. The faster the beat, the more vigorously the arms move. This accounts for the piston-like drive of sprinters. The action is more pendulum-like in distance running. The range of motion is smaller and the arms swing somewhat across the chest, but not past the midline.
- **Hands**. The hands control tension, as you can easily demonstrate to yourself. Hold out your hand, straighten the fingers, and notice the

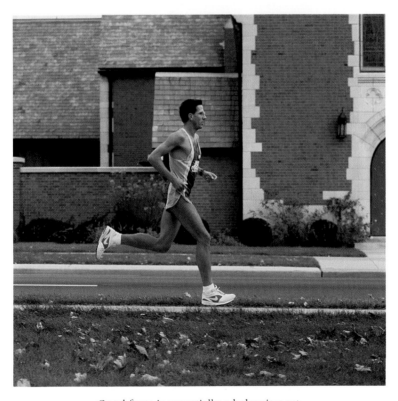

Good form is essentially a balancing act.

feeling of rigidity all the way up your arm. Next, make a fist and clench it tightly. You're tense again, right? Now make a loose fist. Feel better? The unclenched fist, fingers resting lightly on the palms, promotes relaxed running.

- **Wrists**. Moving up the arm, check the wrist. It should be fixed in line with the arms, so hands are not left to flap aimlessly in the breeze.
- **Elbows**. Give careful attention to elbows. They should always be unlocked. Otherwise, you sacrifice the driving and balancing potential of the arms. The arms get their power from the up-and-down motion at elbow level. Try hammering a nail with a stiff elbow, then take advantage of the bend and notice how much more force you generate the second way. Similar forces are at work in running.
- **Shoulders**. The locked elbow also produces one of the most common form faults—a wasteful dipping and swaying motion in the shoulders. Ideally, the shoulders show no apparent movement. They remain parallel to the running surface.

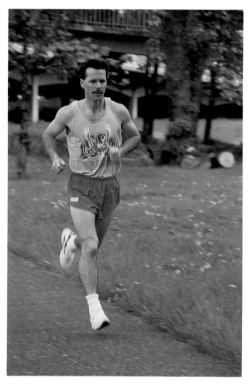

Good posture is an important part of the mix.

Head's Up

You've seen this runner—shuffling around the track with eyes fixed on the feet, and back and shoulders hunched forward in the shape of a number 9.

That's precisely how *not* to run. Straighten up. The best posture for a runner is erect, with the back perpendicular to the ground. The advantages are many: freer use of the legs through a greater range of motion, easier breathing as the unconstricted lungs fill more completely, and a view of something more than your feet.

Tell yourself, Run tall! This means stretching up to your full height, but stopping short of running with the rigid back of a soldier at attention.

Good posture begins just above the hips. Imagine the pelvis as a filled bowl, and try not to spill its contents by leaning forward too much.

The other key to postural control is the head. The gaze of the eyes controls the lean of the body. Look forward, not downward. Cast your eyes on the horizon, and everything else tends to fall into proper alignment.

Smooth, efficient running is also a product of muscle strength and flexibility as well as the body being properly warmed up before the run and cooled down afterward. The next chapter deals with those techniques.

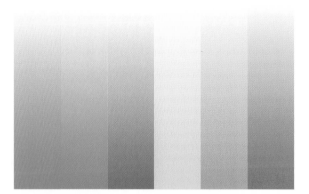

5

Warming Up and Cooling Down

What's the first image that comes to mind when you think of warm-up exercises? It's probably a picture of runners bending and stretching, or perhaps leaning into walls or trees as if trying to push them over.

Such exercises have become a standard tool of running training. If they are done regularly and properly, they keep your stride fluid and they fight off injuries. However, don't confuse these stretching exercises with warming up. They are two separate activities, best done at opposite ends of the run. Warm up by running, walking, or mixing the two. Stretch *after* you run, usually as part of the cool-down period.

Warming to the Task

The best way to warm up for running is by starting with a slow run, or by starting with a fast walk, then breaking into a slow run, and finally slipping into normal pace when your legs and lungs are ready for it.

Listen to your body, the running authorities tell you. Run as you feel. Heed the body's messages, and you'll keep yourself fit and healthy.

Listening isn't enough, however. You must know how to analyze and act upon those signals. You have to realize that the body sometimes tells lies. One of those times is right before you start to run, and this is what makes the warm-up period so critical.

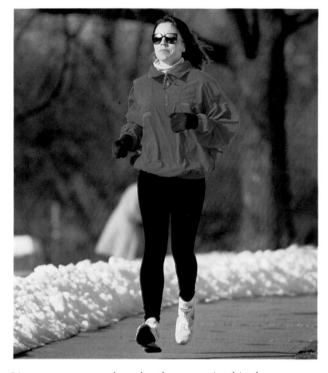

It's up to you to analyze the clues contained in the warm-up.

Let's say for instance, that you're an early-morning runner. You wake up stiff and tired in the chilly predawn. You think, I'm in no shape to run. My body is telling me that I need a day off.

Or perhaps you're a late-afternoon runner. A minor injury has interfered with your recent runs, but you don't notice it while moving through your workday. You think, I'm recovered now and ready for normal running again.

Or let's say you're facing a big race. Your anxiety has you feeling weak and doubtful. You think, Will I even have the strength to get to the starting line?

In each of these scenarios, your body could be lying to you. If you believed everything it said before a run, you'd make a mistake on each of those three days. You might not have run on a morning that could have turned out okay. You might have ignored a minor injury that afternoon and made it major. Or you might have let prerace nerves erode your confidence.

Here's where the warm-up comes in. Besides warming and loosening you physically, this phase of your workout is a truth finder. The warm-up tests your will and ability to run that day. It tells you if you're able to run. It can ease away aches that you thought were serious, or it can uncover those you tried to ignore, or it can chase away your doubts and fears.

The hardest part of running is getting started. Your mind and body rebel against taking the first steps. Ease into your run with those first steps of the warm-up. Plan to walk or run easily for 10 to 20 minutes, roughly the first mile or two. You can integrate the warm-up into the mileage of a long, steady-pace run. Or you can separate it from a faster, timed session and perhaps insert some stretching exercises in between.

By the time you've warmed up, your feelings will be telling the truth. Imaginary or transient problems will have eased if not vanished, and real concerns will still be there, if not intensified.

After you've warmed up is the time to listen closely to your body and to believe what it says. Is it telling you to move on or to back off?

Cooling Down and Stretching Out

The cool-down phase is the warm-up in reverse, with one essential addition afterward—stretching. Just as you warm up with fast walking and easy running to get ready for the harder running to come, you cool down with easy running and walking to shake off the effects of this work. You add stretching to the cool-down to reverse the negative effects of the run.

Your body is in overdrive when you finish running. The harder you ran, the higher its gear is. You may be breathing hard and sweating heavily. At the least, you're warm, your heart is beating at twice its normal rate, and your legs have taken a good pounding. The worst thing you can do to yourself now is jump into your car and drive home. Don't even sit down. Keep moving. Walk briskly or run easily for another 5 to 10 minutes, allowing your pulse and breathing rates to descend gradually toward normal.

Remember that the apparent air temperature rises about 20° while you're running. This will plummet again as soon as you stop, so be prepared to exchange your sweat-soaked shirt for a dry one and to add extra clothing if you'll be outside for long.

Be aware, too, that running is by its nature a tightening activity. It reduces the flexibility in the back of your legs (particularly the calves and hamstrings). If left uncorrected, this tightness sets you up for soreness and injury.

Stretching counteracts the inflexibility that running causes. Therefore, the best time to stretch is after you run, usually during the cool-down period. Another good time to stretch is after the warm-up and before a faster training session or race. Some runners also pause during long road races such as the marathon to work out their tightness.

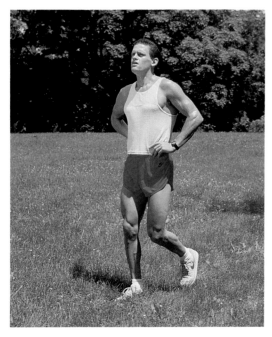

Humor your body—it needs to come down from the run gradually.

The muscles are most receptive to stretching when they're warm and tight, and are least likely to be injured then by the very exercises that are supposed to *prevent* injury. Yes, you read that last line correctly. Stretching exercises can *cause* injuries if done improperly or at the wrong time.

Because the running motion is fast and jarring, the therapeutic stretches need to be slow and soothing. Remember to follow these three key rules of stretching:

1. Stretch *slowly* to the point of discomfort, but do not push or bounce into the pain zone.
2. Breathe normally—don't hold your breath.
3. Once you've found the borderline between comfort and discomfort, hold the exercise at that edge for 10 to 30 seconds.

The rest of this section outlines 10 ways to maintain and regain flexibility. These exercises are designed to counterbalance the tightening effects of running on your muscles.

Note. Stretches and their descriptions are from *Sport Stretch* (pp. 52, 56, 59, 70, 80, 90, 105, 116, 131, 143) by M.J. Alter, Champaign, IL: Leisure Press. Copyright 1990 by Michael J. Alter. Adapted by permission of Human Kinetics.

Plantar Arch

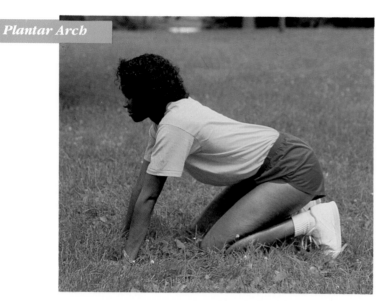

Kneel on all fours with your toes underneath you. Lower your buttocks backward and downward. Hold for 30 seconds.

Ankle

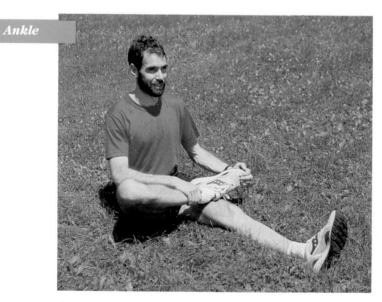

Sit on the floor or ground with your right leg crossed over your left knee. Hold your right ankle or heel with your left hand and slowly pull your foot toward your body. Repeat on the other side.

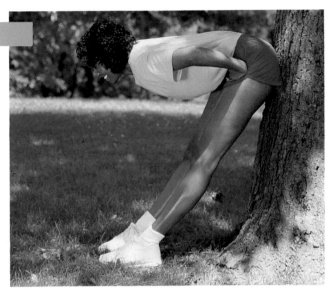

Ankle

Stand with your back flat against a wall or flat surface with your feet 1 or 2 feet away from the surface. Turn your feet slightly inward and slowly lean forward, keeping your legs straight. Hold for 30 seconds.

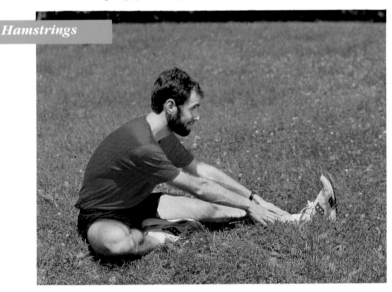

Hamstrings

Sit on the floor or ground with both legs extended in front of you. Bend your right knee and slide your heel toward your crotch. Place your heel against the inner side of your left thigh so that a 90° angle is formed between your extended left leg and flexed right leg. Keeping your left leg straight, bend at the waist, and slowly lower your upper body onto your thigh.

Adductors

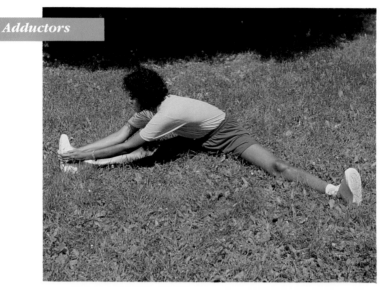

Sit upright on the floor or ground with your legs straddled as much as possible. While keeping your legs extended, bend at the waist, lowering your upper body toward your leg. Repeat on the opposite side.

Quadriceps

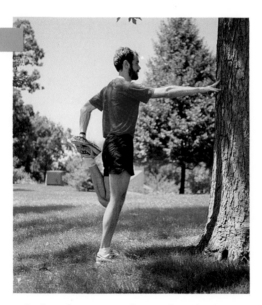

Stand with your right hand against a flat surface for balance and support. Bend your left leg behind you, grasping the foot with your left hand. Slightly flex your right leg and pull your left heel toward your buttocks. Be careful not to over-compress your knee. Repeat with your right leg. Avoid this stretch if you have bad knees.

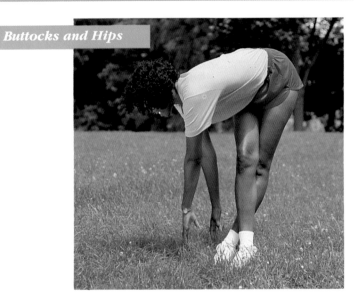

Stand with your hands at your sides. Cross your left leg behind your right leg. Turn to the right, bend at the waist, and try to touch the heel of your left leg with both hands while keeping your legs straight. Hold for 10-20 seconds, then repeat on the opposite side.

Lower Back

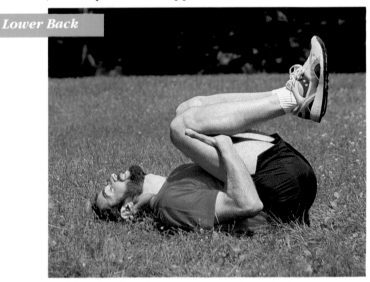

Lie flat on your back. Bend your knees toward your chest, grasping behind your thighs. Pull your knees toward your chest and shoulders until your hips come off the ground. Hold for 10-20 seconds, then extend your legs slowly, one at a time.

Neck

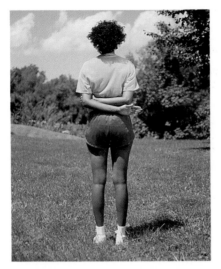

Stand with both arms behind your back. Grasp your left elbow from behind with your right hand. Pull your elbow across the midline of your back, and tilt your head toward your right shoulder, keeping your left shoulder flat. Repeat on the opposite side.

Shoulders

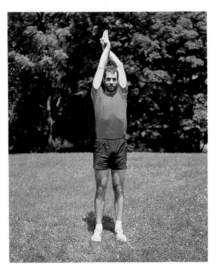

While standing, raise both arms over your head. Cross one wrist over the other and interlock your hands. Straighten your arms and stretch upward.

You've now completed the tour of the running perimeter. You know what to do before and after you run—now it's time to take the plunge into our recommended workouts.

PART II

RUNNING WORKOUT ZONES

This book takes a unique approach to categorizing workouts. We place them in color-coded zones according to each workout's duration and intensity. The workouts are distributed across the zones according to level of difficulty. Green training is the easiest, then come the Blue, Purple, Yellow, and Orange zones with steadily increasing degrees of difficulty. Red workouts are the hardest.

Workouts progress in difficulty through the zone. The first is the least demanding and the last the most demanding. The duration of workouts is determined by how many minutes they take to complete. Thirty minutes is our dividing line between shorter and longer runs. Intensity is determined either by actual running pace or by how hard the run feels. The hardest workouts are timed for speed, while in others intensity is rated in terms of how the workouts feel.

WORKOUT COLOR ZONES			
Zone (chapter)	Type of workout	RPE	Time
Green (6)	Low intensity, short duration	1-4	<30 min
Blue (7)	Low intensity, long duration	1-4	>30 min
Purple (8)	Medium intensity, short duration	5-7	<30 min
Yellow (9)	Medium intensity, long duration	5-7	>30 min
Orange (10)	High intensity, short duration	8-10	<30 min
Red (11)	High intensity, long duration	8-10	>30 min

Perceived Exertion

Listen to your body, the fitness authorities tell you. It will tell you how hard it is working, and how hard it can work. This can be done by computing percentages of maximum heart rate. Many fitness programs are based on these readings, which are valid measures of effort.

You can stop periodically and check your pulse, then figure how close to maximum you are or should be running. Or you can buy a heart-rate monitor to do the counting for you.

Or you can simply ask yourself, How do I feel? Most runners already do this. They talk about how easy or hard a run is. We simply ask you to take the next step by scoring the degree of difficulty.

Dr. Gunnar Borg found that a person's sense of how difficult running feels lines up very closely with objective measurements of exertion, such as percentages of maximum heart rate and $\dot{V}O_2$max. Dr. Borg originally devised a 20-point scale of rating of perceived exertion to identify these levels of intensity.

Borg and Dr. Bruce Noble later revised the RPE to a scale of 10. We use that improved version here (see Table II.1). The easiest running would rate one point on the Borg-Noble scale, while 10 would be the most strenuous running you could tolerate.

For reference, we've listed the approximate percentages of maximum pulse rate that correspond with each RPE level. The easiest way to estimate your top pulse is to subtract your age from 220:

$$\text{max HR} = 220 - \text{your age}$$

If you're 20 years old, your heart rate peaks at about 200 beats per minute. If you're 40, it peaks at about 180.

However, in many of the workouts, your innate perception of effort is the guiding factor, not heart rate or timed pace. Borg and Noble use the terms *weak*, *moderate*, and *strong* to describe intensities. We translate these levels to *low*, *medium*, and *high* in our system.

Table II.1 How Hard It Feels		
RPE	**Perception of effort**	**Heart rate**
1	Minimum intensity	<60%
2 & 3	Low intensity	60-69%
4	Low-medium intensity	70-74%
5 & 6	Medium intensity	75-84%
7	Medium-high intensity	85-89%
8 & 9	High intensity	90-99%
10	Maximum intensity	100%

Note. From G.A. Borg's "Psychophysical bases of perceived exertion," *Medicine and Science in Sports and Exercise*, Volume 14, pp. 337-387. Copyright 1982 by the American College of Sports Medicine. Adapted by permission of Williams and Wilkins.

Green and Blue workouts carry an RPE score of 1 to 4. Purple and Yellow workouts are 5 to 7. Orange and Red workouts earn scores of 8 to 10.

Caloric Cost

Running is an energy burner par excellence. Weight-conscious runners like to know about how many kilocalories (kcal) they burn. Table II.2 is based on the color-coded workout zones.

We can't be precise here but we can give fairly accurate estimates. They're based on a 150-pound runner. Add 10% to these totals for each 15 pounds over 150, and subtract 10% for each 15 pounds under 150.

A 150-pound man who runs a Blue workout lasting 40 minutes would burn 400 calories:

$$10 \text{ kcal per minute} \times 40 \text{ minutes} = 400 \text{ kcal}$$

A 135-pound woman who runs the same workout would burn 360 calories:

$$400 \text{ kcal} - (.10 \times 400 \text{ kcal}) = 360 \text{ kcal}$$

Table II.2
Caloric Costs of Running

Zone	Kcal/min	Workout	Total kcals*
Green	10	<30 min	<300
Blue	10	>30 min	>300
Purple	15	<30 min	<450
Yellow	15	>30 min	>450
Orange	20	<30 min	<600
Red	20	>30 min	>600

*Doing the recommended warm-up and cool-down periods will increase the amount of calorie-burning in all zones.

Determining Distance

Most Americans still train by mile distances, but competitive running is an increasingly metric sport. So this is a "bilingual" book. We put most of the training in mile terms, and most of the racing in kilometers.

One kilometer (commonly referred to as a *K*) equals 1000 meters or 62% of a mile. One mile is 1609 meters, a 5-mile run is 8.05 kilometers, and 10 miles is 16.1 kilometers. The marathon equals 26.22 miles or 42.19 kilometers. Table II.3 lists yard/mile equivalents for various metric distances.

Remember that standard outdoor running tracks measure either a quarter-mile (440 yards) or 400 meters per lap. The difference in yard and metric lap times amounts to only a fraction of a second.

We take a cookbook approach to running training in the remainder of this fitness book. In cooking, you achieve satisfying results by combining quality ingredients for proven recipes. The same is true here. First, we familiarize you with the remaining ingredients by describing them completely in Part II. Then we give you recipes for successful running in Part III. The raw materials take the form of individual workouts. Dozens of them make up chapters 6 to 11.

Table II.3
Metric Distances

Metric distance	Yard/mile equivalent
50 meters	54.68 yards
100 meters	109.36 yards
150 meters	164.04 yards
200 meters	218.72 yards
300 meters	328.08 yards
400 meters	437.44 yards
500 meters	526.81 yards
600 meters	656.17 yards
800 meters	874.88 yards
1000 meters	1093.61 yards
1200 meters	1312.33 yards
1500 meters	1640.33 yards
3 kilometers	1.86 miles
5 kilometers	3.11 miles
8 kilometers	4.97 miles
10 kilometers	6.21 miles
12 kilometers	7.46 miles
15 kilometers	9.32 miles
20 kilometers	12.43 miles
25 kilometers	15.54 miles
30 kilometers	18.64 miles
40 kilometers	24.86 miles

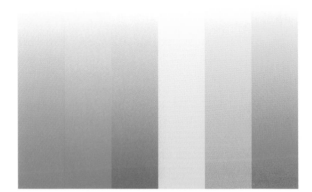

Green Zone

Greens are your easiest workouts, being both low in intensity and relatively short. They carry a rating of perceived exertion (RPE) in the 1 to 4 range, last less than 30 minutes, and cover distances of 1 to 3 miles.

The 10 Green workouts are adaptable to all types of runners and their varying needs. They fulfill the basic exercise requirements, let you ease down your training before hard efforts, help you recover from those big efforts, and even inject a low-key form of speed training.

This chapter introduces you to three types of runs:

- **Easy.** This is your most basic run, one of your shortest and certainly the least intense. You simply find a pace that is comfortable, then maintain it for the duration.

  This instruction may mean running slowly all the way if you're a seasoned runner or mixing in some walking if you're new to the activity. Either way, it should not be a challenging session.

  The easy run is a staple of the beginning-running programs in this book. But it also works well as a break from harder training in the frequent running and competitive running programs. It lets you maintain basic fitness without overly taxing yourself.

- **Steady.** You'll maintain a steady pace throughout this run. The workout may be a little longer than the easy run, but the key difference is that it is somewhat faster.

At lower intensities, steady runs serve the same purposes as easy ones while being a tad more demanding. They remain well within the reach of an exercise runner.

At higher intensities, steady runs are part of the breaking-in process for timed workouts and races. Here, they do the most good for frequent runners and competitive runners.

- **Fartlek**. This Swedish word means *speed play*, which rather accurately describes the practice. It is a relaxed form of interval training, which we'll introduce fully in chapter 8.

Basically, interval workouts usually are run on a track. They alternate short, fast segments of running with slow, easy recovery periods according to a predetermined plan.

The pace also alternates between fast and slow in fartlek runs. The main difference is that fartlek lacks the formal structure of intervals. Accelerations are done by whim rather than by plan, and the running is most often done outside the confines of a track.

The major benefit of fartlek training for all runners is breaking you out of a one-pace rut. Fartlek works you through a wider range of physical motion than easy or steady runs do, and it gives a true mental change of pace to your program.

Fartlek also serves as an unpressured form of speedwork for runners who are preparing to race. It's a transition to and a break from formal, timed interval workouts on the track.

WORKOUT 1

EASY RUN
TOTAL TIME: 20-25 minutes

1

WARM-UP: Walk about 5 minutes.

WORKOUT
Distance: 1 mile
Time: 7-11 minutes
Pace: 7-11 minutes per mile
Effort: RPE 2-4
% max HR: 60-74

COOL-DOWN: Walk about 5 minutes, then stretch.

CALORIES BURNED: 200-250

COMMENTS

This workout is used primarily by beginning runners; others find it too short. A beginner may take brief walking breaks if necessary to complete the mile. For example, you might run a quarter-mile, walk a minute, run another quarter-mile, and so on. Walking is perfectly acceptable, but don't count it in your total distance. Make the running add up to 1 mile, which most runners complete in 7 to 10 minutes.

WORKOUT 2

2

EASY RUN
TOTAL TIME: 30-35 minutes

WARM-UP: Walk about 5 minutes.

WORKOUT
Distance: 2 miles
Time: 14-22 minutes
Pace: 7-11 minutes per mile
Effort: RPE 2-4
   % max HR: 60-74

COOL-DOWN: Walk about 5 minutes, then stretch.

CALORIES BURNED: 300-350

COMMENTS
Don't try this workout until you can comfortably complete Green Workout 1 without walking. It's okay to take walking breaks in Workout 2, as long as the running still totals 2 miles.

WORKOUT 3

EASY RUN
TOTAL TIME: 35-45 minutes

3

WARM-UP: Walk about 5 minutes.

WORKOUT
Distance: 3 miles
Time: 21-33 minutes
Pace: 7-11 minutes per mile
Effort: RPE 2-4
   % max HR: 60-74

COOL-DOWN: Walk about 5 minutes, then stretch.

CALORIES BURNED: 350-450

COMMENTS
Wait to try this workout until you can complete Green Workout 2 without walking. Take walk breaks in Workout 3 if necessary as long as your running still totals 3 miles.

WORKOUT 4

STEADY RUN
TOTAL TIME: 25-30 minutes

WARM-UP: Walk and/or run easily for 5-10 minutes.

WORKOUT
Distance: 1 mile
Time: 6-10 minutes
Pace: 6-10 minutes per mile
Effort: RPE 3-4
% max HR: 65-74

COOL-DOWN: Walk about 5 minutes, then stretch.

CALORIES BURNED: 250-300

COMMENTS

Run slightly faster in this workout than in the easy runs, but still keep the intensity in the low range. Include no walking breaks. If you need them, you shouldn't be trying this workout yet. Faster runners need to include easy running in their warm-up.

WORKOUT 5

STEADY RUN
TOTAL TIME: 30-40 minutes

5

WARM-UP: Walk and/or run easily for 5-10 minutes.

WORKOUT

Distance: 2 miles

Time: 12-20 minutes

Pace: 6-10 minutes per mile

Effort: RPE 3-4

% max HR: 65-74

COOL-DOWN: Walk about 5 minutes, then stretch.

CALORIES BURNED: 300-400

COMMENTS

Don't try this workout until you can finish a 1-mile steady run without struggling.

WORKOUT 6

STEADY RUN
TOTAL TIME: 40-50 minutes

WARM-UP: Walk and/or run easily for 5-10 minutes.

WORKOUT

Distance: 3 miles
Time: 18-30 minutes
Pace: 6-10 minutes per mile
Effort: RPE 3-4
    % max HR: 65-74

COOL-DOWN: Walk about 5 minutes, then stretch.

CALORIES BURNED: 400-500

COMMENTS

Wait to try this workout after you've completed a 2-mile steady run.

WORKOUT 7

STEADY RUN
TOTAL TIME: 45-50 minutes

7

WARM-UP: Walk at start, then run easily for 5-10 minutes.

WORKOUT

Distance: 4 miles

Time: 24-30 minutes

Pace: Under 7-1/2 minutes per mile

Effort: RPE 3-4
% max HR: 65-74

COOL-DOWN: Walk about 5 minutes, then stretch.

CALORIES BURNED: 450-500

COMMENTS

This workout is reserved for runners who can complete the 4 miles in 30 minutes or less. Try it only if you can average 7-1/2 minutes per mile or faster. Otherwise, consider it a Blue-zone Workout.

WORKOUT 8

8

FARTLEK RUN
TOTAL TIME: 25-30 minutes

WARM-UP: Walk and/or run easily for 5-10 minutes.

WORKOUT

Distance: 1 mile
Time: 7-11 minutes
Pace: Varied, averaging 7-11 minutes per mile
Effort: Average RPE 4 (2-6 range)
      % max HR: 60-84

COOL-DOWN: Walk about 5 minutes, then stretch.

CALORIES BURNED: 250-300

COMMENTS

Emphasize varying your pace. Divide the distance into segments and run them at different efforts. For example, run easily for the first quarter-mile, then accelerate to high speed for a hundred yards or so, run easily for another quarter-mile to recover, shift to a faster steady pace for a few hundred yards, and kick into a higher gear to finish.

WORKOUT 9

FARTLEK RUN
TOTAL TIME: 35-40 minutes

9

WARM-UP: Walk and/or run easily for 5-10 minutes.

WORKOUT
Distance: 2 miles
Time: 14-22 minutes
Pace: Varied, averaging 7-11 minutes per mile
Effort: Average RPE 4 (2-6 range)
% max HR: 60-84

COOL-DOWN: Walk about 5 minutes, then stretch.

CALORIES BURNED: 350-400

COMMENTS
Try this workout only after you have finished a 1-mile fartlek run without struggling.

10

FARTLEK RUN
TOTAL TIME: 40-50 minutes

WARM-UP: Walk and/or run easily for 5-10 minutes.

WORKOUT

Distance: 3 miles

Time: 21-33 minutes

Pace: Varied, averaging 7-11 minutes per mile

Effort: Average RPE 4 (2-6 range)
% max HR: 60-84

COOL-DOWN: Walk about 5 minutes, then stretch.

CALORIES BURNED: 400-500

COMMENTS

Save this workout until you've had a successful 2-mile fartlek run.

Workout	Description	Duration	Distance	Intensity
		Summary Table		
		Green Zone Workouts		
1	Easy run	7-10 minutes	1 mile	RPE: 2-4 % max HR: 60-74
2	Easy run	14-20 minutes	2 miles	RPE: 2-4 % max HR: 60-74
3	Easy run	21-30 minutes	3 miles	RPE: 2-4 % max HR: 60-74
4	Steady run	6-10 minutes	1 mile	RPE: 3-4 % max HR: 65-74
5	Steady run	12-20 minutes	2 miles	RPE: 3-4 % max HR: 65-74
6	Steady run	18-30 minutes	3 miles	RPE: 3-4 % max HR: 65-74
7	Steady run	24-30 minutes	4 miles	RPE: 3-4 % max HR: 65-74
8	Fartlek run	7-10 minutes	1 mile	RPE: 4 (average) % max HR: 60-84
9	Fartlek run	14-20 minutes	2 miles	RPE: 4 (average) % max HR: 60-84
10	Fartlek run	21-30 minutes	3 miles	RPE: 4 (average) % max HR: 60-84

Longer-duration versions of these low-intensity workouts appear in the next chapter, the Blue zone.

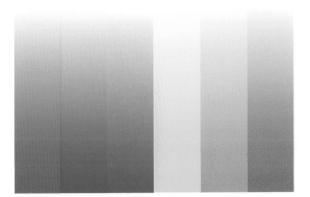

Blue Zone

Blues are similar in content and effort to workouts in the Green zone, and offer the same benefits. Blues still fall into the rating of perceived exertion (RPE) range of 1 to 4. In other words, they're rather easy.

However, Blue workouts last longer than Greens, with 30 minutes now becoming the *lower* rather than the upper limit. The distances covered will usually top 4 miles.

The 10 Blue workouts remain within reach of most runners, regardless of whether you place yourself in the beginning, frequent, or competitive class. Your current training level will determine if the longest distances offered in this chapter are within your reach or interest.

We introduce you to a new type of workout in this chapter: the long run. As the name suggests, this run is longer than any of the easy or steady runs. You run long at a comfortable pace, one that allows you to enjoy the scenery and lets your mind wander. You don't force the pace.

WORKOUT 1

1

EASY RUN
TOTAL TIME: 45-55 minutes

WARM-UP: Walk about 5 minutes (optional).

WORKOUT
Distance: 4 miles
Time: 30-44 minutes
Pace: 7-11 minutes per mile
Effort: RPE 2-4
% max HR: 60-74

COOL-DOWN: Walk about 5 minutes, then stretch.

CALORIES BURNED: 450-500

COMMENTS

Walk at the start if you feel tight. But usually you can incorporate the warm-up into this workout by running very easily for the first mile or so.

WORKOUT 2

EASY RUN

TOTAL TIME: 45 minutes to 1 hour, 5 minutes

2

WARM-UP: Walk about 5 minutes (optional).

WORKOUT
Distance: 5 miles
Time: 35-55 minutes
Pace: 7-11 minutes per mile
Effort: RPE 2-4
% max HR: 60-74

COOL-DOWN: Walk about 5 minutes, then stretch.

CALORIES BURNED: 450-650

COMMENTS
Your effort should remain easy throughout this run, but your pace may vary. You typically will start at a slower–than–average pace before you're warmed up, and finish a little faster as you get into the flow of the run.

WORKOUT 3

3

EASY RUN
TOTAL TIME: 55 minutes to 1 hour, 15 minutes

WARM-UP: Walk about 5 minutes (optional).

WORKOUT

Distance: 6 miles

Time: 42 minutes to 1 hour, 6 minutes

Pace: 7-11 minutes per mile

Effort: RPE 2-4

% max HR: 60-74

COOL-DOWN: Walk about 5 minutes, then stretch.

CALORIES BURNED: 550-650

COMMENTS

If the 6-mile workout takes you an hour or more to finish, consider this a long run. An hour's running pushes the effort beyond easy.

WORKOUT 4

STEADY RUN
TOTAL TIME: 40 minutes to 1 hour, 5 minutes

4

WARM-UP: Walk or run easily for 5-10 minutes (optional).

WORKOUT

Distance: 5 miles
Time: 30-50 minutes
Pace: 6-10 minutes per mile
Effort: RPE 3-4
% max HR: 65-74

COOL-DOWN: Walk about 5 minutes, then stretch.

CALORIES BURNED: 400-650

COMMENTS

Because the pace is slightly faster in steady runs than in easy runs, you may now need more warm-up. Take the walk and/or slower run separately, or run easily for the first mile of your steady run.

WORKOUT 5

5

STEADY RUN
TOTAL TIME: 45 minutes to 1 hour, 15 minutes

WARM-UP: Walk or run easily for 5-10 minutes (optional).

WORKOUT
Distance: 6 miles
Time: 36 minutes to 1 hour
Pace: 6-10 minutes per mile
Effort: RPE 3-4
% max HR: 65-74

COOL-DOWN: Walk about 5 minutes, then stretch.

CALORIES BURNED: 450-750

COMMENTS
For reasons given in Blue Workout 3, the steady 6-mile run is reserved for runners who can complete this distance in well under an hour.

WORKOUT 6

LONG RUN
TOTAL TIME: 1 hour to 1 hour, 25 minutes

6

WARM-UP: Incorporate into the workout as a very slowly paced first mile or so.

WORKOUT
Distance: 7 miles
Time: 49 minutes to 1 hour, 17 minutes
Pace: 7-11 minutes per mile
Effort: RPE 3-4
% max HR: 65-74

COOL-DOWN: Walk about 5 minutes, then stretch.

CALORIES BURNED: 600-800

COMMENTS
If you think you'll have trouble running this distance nonstop, insert walking breaks. For example, run a mile, then walk a minute or two, and so on. Don't count the walking toward your total distance.

WORKOUT 7

7

LONG RUN
TOTAL TIME: 1 hour, 5 minutes to 1 hour, 35 minutes

WARM-UP: Incorporate into the long run as a very slowly paced first mile or so.

WORKOUT
Distance: 8 miles
Time: 56 minutes to 1 hour, 28 minutes
Pace: 7-11 minutes per mile
Effort: RPE 3-4
      % max HR: 65-74

COOL-DOWN: Walk about 5 minutes, then stretch.

CALORIES BURNED: 650-900

COMMENTS
The longer your run, the more time you'll need to recover from it no matter how slowly you run. Be sure to schedule at least one rest day after your long run.

WORKOUT 8

LONG RUN
TOTAL TIME: 1 hour, 15 minutes to 1 hour, 45 minutes

8

WARM-UP: Incorporate into the long run as a very slowly paced first mile or so.

WORKOUT

Distance: 9 miles

Time: 1 hour, 3 minutes to 1 hour, 40 minutes

Pace: 7-11 minutes per mile

Effort: RPE 3-4

% max HR: 65-74

COOL-DOWN: Walk about 5 minutes, then stretch.

CALORIES BURNED: 750-1,000

COMMENTS

Your total time commitment for this workout is about 1-1/2 hours. Schedule it on a weekend or holiday when you have the most free time.

WORKOUT 9

9

FARTLEK RUN
TOTAL TIME: 50 minutes to 1 hour

WARM-UP: Walk and/or run easily for 5-10 minutes.

WORKOUT
Distance: 4 miles
Time: 30-44 minutes
Pace: Varied, averaging 7-11 minutes per mile
Effort: Average RPE 4 (2-6 range)
% max HR: 60-84

COOL-DOWN: Walk about 5 minutes, then stretch.

CALORIES BURNED: 500-600

COMMENTS
Attempt this workout only if your slower easy, steady, or long workouts are significantly longer than your faster-paced fartlek run.

WORKOUT 10

FARTLEK RUN
TOTAL TIME: 55 minutes to 1 hour, 10 minutes

10

WARM-UP: Walk and/or run easily for 5-10 minutes.

WORKOUT

Distance: 5 miles

Time: 35-55 minutes

Pace: Varied, averaging 7-11 minutes per mile

Effort: Average RPE 4 (2-6 range)
       % max HR: 60-84

COOL-DOWN: Walk about 5 minutes, then stretch.

CALORIES BURNED: 550-700

COMMENTS

If you already run races or plan to race anytime soon, make sure that some portion of the fartlek run reaches your maximum racing pace.

| | | Summary Table | | |
| | | Blue Zone Workouts | | |
Workout	Description	Duration	Distance	Intensity
1	Easy run	30-40 minutes	4 miles	RPE: 2-4 % max HR: 60-74
2	Easy run	35-50 minutes	5 miles	RPE: 2-4 % max HR: 60-74
3	Easy run	42-60 minutes	6 miles	RPE: 2-4 % max HR: 60-74
4	Steady run	30-50 minutes	5 miles	RPE: 3-4 % max HR: 65-74
5	Steady run	36-60 minutes	6 miles	RPE: 3-4 % max HR: 65-74
6	Long run	49-70 minutes	7 miles	RPE: 3-4 % max HR: 65-74
7	Long run	56-80 minutes	8 miles	RPE: 3-4 % max HR: 65-74
8	Long run	63-90 minutes	9 miles	RPE: 3-4 % max HR: 65-74
9	Fartlek run	30-40 minutes	4 miles	RPE: 4 (average) % max HR: 60-84
10	Fartlek run	35-50 minutes	5 miles	RPE: 4 (average) % max HR: 60-84

This completes your low-intensity workouts. Next, the difficulty level steps up to medium in the Purple zone.

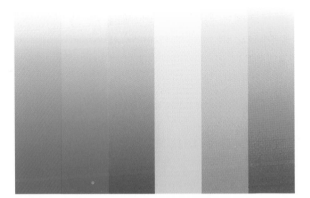

8

Purple Zone

Purple workouts increase in intensity compared to those in the Green and Blue zones. Purples carry a rating of perceived exertion (RPE) in the 5 to 7 range. They last less than 30 minutes, and the distances covered are typically 1 to 3 miles.

The 10 Purple workouts occupy a middle range between easy and hard, and they take some of their elements from both directions. You're given somewhat more intense steady and fartlek runs, yet you also receive a more modest version of speedwork than you'll find in later zones.

Medium-intensity runs are valuable to anyone who wants to break through to a new performance level, or merely to inject more variety into the routine. They're vital workouts for anyone who plans to run races, with Purples geared to racing at 5 kilometer or shorter distances.

Date Pace and Goal Pace

Many of the runs now will be timed for speed. In these sessions, you need to know the running pace that's best for you. So we introduce the concepts of date pace (DP) and goal pace (GP).

DP is the pace you could run now for a selected distance. GP is the pace that you would realistically like to run 8 to 10 months from now.

DP might be determined by the result of a recent 12-minute test (see chapter 3). This would determine your current reading for $\dot{V}O_2$max. A realistic GP would be two $\dot{V}O_2$ levels higher on Table 3.1. For example, your latest 12-minute test gives you a current $\dot{V}O_2$ reading of 42.2. You can expect to reach a goal of 46.1 over the next several months.

Looking ahead to chapter 12, we can tell you what these figures mean in terms of a 10-kilometer race. Your DP for 10K is 47:16 or 7:36 per mile. Your realistic goal is 43:49 or 7:04 per mile.

Interval Training

You'll use date pace and goal pace while running intervals. Interval training is basic to any effective training program. It involves shorter, faster runs that are repeated several times with appropriate periods of recovery between runs. Intervals are usually run at about the pace of a particular race distance.

Intervals have several benefits. The first, obviously, is to teach pace judgment. Most of these workouts are timed, so you learn how it feels to run at a particular tempo.

Physically, the intervals prepare you for the fastest pace you'll encounter in a race. They help immunize you against the stresses to the legs and lungs that you'll inevitably encounter as the intensity increases.

Intervals also let you do more work intermittently than you could do continuously. In other words, you can run 12 individual laps on a track at higher speed than you could run 3 miles without recovery breaks. Or you can cover more total distance interval-style than you could run steadily at the same pace.

Intervals may vary in length from less than 100 meters to more than a mile, and are most commonly run on a track. The recovery between intervals may be accomplished by jogging or walking. We recommend a jog or walk of equal distance to the fast interval for distances up to 800 meters, and 800 meters for all longer distances. In the workouts, a walk or jog of 100 meters will be referred to as a "walk/jog 100."

The amount of running (excluding warm-up, cool-down, and recovery periods) in our interval-training workouts generally totals 1 to 3 miles, but sometimes extends longer. A warm-up period precedes all interval workouts, and a cool-down follows.

An easy warm-up run of 1 to 2 miles should precede interval sessions. Finish warming up with strides—running 100 meters 4 to 6 times.

These short-distance strides complete your preparation for the full-scale speed workout that follows. The pace of the strides increases with each one, until the last is slightly faster than the first interval in the main workout.

Finish the interval session with a cool-down. This again should be an easy 1- to 2-mile run.

This chapter leads you into four subcategories of interval workouts:

- **Goal-pace/date-pace intervals**. This workout alternates between repetitions at GP and at DP.
- **Goal-pace intervals**. This workout is run almost entirely at GP and has fewer repetitions.
- **Underdistance intervals**. These are shorter than your racing distance and are run at the DP for that racing distance.
- **Rhythm intervals**. These are short, continuous intervals without a normal jog-walk recovery period. The pace alternates between GP and one significantly slower than DP (during which some recovery occurs).

WORKOUT 1

1

STEADY RUN
TOTAL TIME: 30-40 minutes

WARM-UP: Run an easy mile or so, then walk a few minutes before starting main workout.

WORKOUT

Distance: 2 miles

Time: 12-20 minutes

Pace: 6-10 minutes per mile

Effort: RPE 5
% max HR: 75-79

COOL-DOWN: Walk a few minutes, then run an easy mile or so, walk again, and stretch.

CALORIES BURNED: 300-400

COMMENTS

As the pace of your workouts becomes faster in this zone, you build into them and ease down from them with an additional slow mile or more in the warm-up and again in the cool-down.

WORKOUT 2

STEADY RUN
TOTAL TIME: 35-50 minutes

2

WARM-UP: Run an easy mile or so, then walk a few minutes before starting main workout.

WORKOUT

Distance: 3 miles
Time: 18-30 minutes
Pace: 6-10 minutes per mile
Effort: RPE 5
      % max HR: 75-79

COOL-DOWN: Walk a few minutes, then run an easy mile or so, walk again, and stretch.

CALORIES BURNED: 350-500

COMMENTS

The steady runs are transitional workouts between the easy ones of the earlier chapters and the race-like efforts to come. Steady runs take you out of your comfort zone, but not as far out as will the workouts in later chapters.

WORKOUT 3

3

STEADY RUN
TOTAL TIME: 45-55 minutes

WARM-UP: Run an easy mile or so, then walk a few minutes before starting main workout.

WORKOUT
Distance: 4 miles
Time: 24-30 minutes
Pace: Under 7-1/2 minutes per mile
Effort: RPE 5
% max HR: 75-79

COOL-DOWN: Walk a few minutes, then run an easy mile or so, walk again, and stretch.

CALORIES BURNED: 450-550

COMMENTS
This workout is intended only for runners who can finish the 4 miles in 30 minutes or less. Skip it if you can't average 7-1/2 minutes per mile or faster.

WORKOUT 4

FARTLEK RUN
TOTAL TIME: 30-40 minutes

4

WARM-UP: Run an easy mile or so, then walk a few minutes before starting main workout.

WORKOUT

Distance: 2 miles
Time: 14-20 minutes
Pace: Varied, averaging 7-10 minutes per mile
Effort: Average RPE 6 (2-10 range)
% max HR: 60-100

COOL-DOWN: Walk a few minutes, then run an easy mile or so, walk again, and stretch.

CALORIES BURNED: 300-400

COMMENTS

Note the higher level of effort than you've experienced in previous fartlek runs. The bursts of speed may now be either longer or faster, sometimes briefly reaching maximum RPE of 10 for the first time in our series of workouts.

5

FARTLEK RUN
TOTAL TIME: 35-45 minutes

WARM-UP: Run an easy mile or so, then walk a few minutes before starting main workout.

WORKOUT

Distance: 3 miles

Time: 21-30 minutes

Pace: Varied, averaging 7-10 minutes per mile

Effort: Average RPE 6 (2-10 range)
% max HR: 60-100

COOL-DOWN: Walk a few minutes, then run an easy mile or so, walk again, and stretch.

CALORIES BURNED: 350-450

COMMENTS

A reminder that fartlek should be anything but evenly paced running. At best, it's an all-in-one workout with paces ranging all the way from jogging to sprinting.

WORKOUT 6

FARTLEK RUN
TOTAL TIME: 45-50 minutes

6

WARM-UP: Run an easy mile or so, then walk a few minutes before starting main workout.

WORKOUT

Distance: 4 miles

Time: 28-30 minutes

Pace: Varied, averaging under 7-1/2 minutes per mile

Effort: Average RPE 6 (2-10 range)
% max HR: 60-100

COOL-DOWN: Walk a few minutes, then run an easy mile or so, walk again, and stretch.

CALORIES BURNED: 450-500

COMMENTS

Do this workout only if you can finish the 4 fartlek miles in a half-hour or less, or average 7-1/2 minutes per mile or faster.

WORKOUT 7

7

GOAL-PACE/DATE-PACE INTERVALS
TOTAL TIME: 40 minutes to 1 hour

WARM-UP: Run an easy mile or 2, walk a few minutes, then take 4 to 6 100-meter strides with walk-jog 100s between, and walk again before starting main workout.

WORKOUT

Distance: Fast segments total 1-3 miles.

Recovery: Walk or jog equal distance between intervals 800 meters and shorter, and stay at 800 walk-jog for longer intervals.

Time: Fast segments total 30 minutes or less.

Pace: Mix goal pace and date pace for your chosen distance.

Effort: RPE 5-7
% max HR: 75-89

COOL-DOWN: Walk a few minutes, then run an easy mile or 2, walk again, and stretch.

CALORIES BURNED: 400-600

COMMENTS

Goal-pace/date-pace interval workout for a mile runner might be 2 x 400 meters at GP with 400 walk-jogs between; 2 × 400 at DP with 400s between. Total distance of fast segments is 1600 meters, or about 1 mile.

WORKOUT 8

GOAL-PACE INTERVALS
TOTAL TIME: 40 minutes to 1 hour

8

WARM-UP: Run an easy mile or two, walk a few minutes, then take 4 to 6 100-meter strides with walk-jog 100s between, and walk again before starting main workout.

WORKOUT

Distance: Fast segments total 1-3 miles.

Recovery: Walk or jog equal distance between intervals 800 meters and shorter, and stay at 800 walk-jog for longer intervals.

Time: Fast segments total 30 minutes or less.

Pace: Goal pace for your chosen distance

Effort: RPE 5-7
    % max HR: 75-89

COOL-DOWN: Walk a few minutes, then run an easy mile or 2, walk again, and stretch.

CALORIES BURNED: 400-600

COMMENTS

Goal-pace interval workout for a 5000-meter runner might be 4 × 1000 meters at GP with 800 walk-jogs between. Total distance of fast segments is 4000 meters, or about 2.5 miles.

WORKOUT 9

9 UNDERDISTANCE INTERVALS
TOTAL TIME: 40 minutes to 1 hour

WARM-UP: Run an easy mile or 2, walk a few minutes, then take 4 to 6 100-meter strides with walk-jog 100s between, and walk again before starting main workout.

WORKOUT

Distance: Fast segments total 1-3 miles.

Recovery: Walk or jog equal distance between intervals 800 meters and shorter, and stay at 800 walk-jog for longer intervals.

Time: Fast segments total 30 minutes or less.

Pace: Date pace for your chosen distance.

Effort: RPE 5-7
  % max HR: 75-89

COOL-DOWN: Walk a few minutes, then run an easy mile or 2, walk again, and stretch.

CALORIES BURNED: 400-600

COMMENTS

Underdistance interval workout for a mile runner might be 1200 meters at DP, walk-jog 800, 600 at DP, walk-jog 600. Total distance of fast segments is 1800 meters, or about 1.2 miles.

WORKOUT 10

RHYTHM INTERVALS
TOTAL TIME: 40 minutes to 1 hour

10

WARM-UP: Run an easy mile or 2, walk a few minutes, then take 4 to 6 100-meter strides with walk-jog 100s between, and walk again before starting main workout.

WORKOUT

Distance: Fast segments total 1-3 miles.

Recovery: Dispense with normal walk-jog recovery segments; entire workout is fast.

Time: Fast segments total 30 minutes or less.

Pace: Alternate between intervals run at goal pace and somewhat slower than date pace.

Effort: RPE 5-7
% max HR:75-89

COOL-DOWN: Walk a few minutes, then run an easy mile or 2, walk again, and end with stretching.

CALORIES BURNED: 400-600

COMMENTS

Rhythm interval workout for a 5000-meter runner might be 12 × 400 meters with 6 of the intervals at GP alternating with 6 at slower than DP. Total distance for fast segments is 4800 meters, or about 3 miles.

Summary Table Purple Zone Workouts				
Workout	**Description**	**Duration**	**Distance**	**Intensity**
1	Steady run	12-20 minutes	2 miles	RPE: 5 % max HR: 75-79
2	Steady run	18-30 minutes	3 miles	RPE: 5 % max HR: 75-79
3	Steady run	24-30 minutes	4 miles	RPE: 5 % max HR: 75-79
4	Fartlek run	14-20 minutes	2 miles	RPE: 6 (average) % max HR: 60-100
5	Fartlek run	21-30 minutes	3 miles	RPE: 6 (average) % max HR: 60-100
6	Fartlek run	28-30 minutes	4 miles	RPE: 6 (average) % max HR: 60-100
7	GP/DP intervals	30 minutes or less	1-3 miles	RPE: 5-7 % max HR: 75-89
8	GP intervals	30 minutes or less	1-3 miles	RPE: 5-7 % max HR: 75-89
9	UD intervals	30 minutes or less	1-3 miles	RPE: 5-7 % max HR: 75-89
10	Rhythm intervals	30 minutes or less	1-3 miles	RPE: 5-7 % max HR: 75-89

Some of these workouts will appear again in longer form in the next chapter's Yellow zone. Others will reemerge in chapter 10 as greater-intensity Oranges.

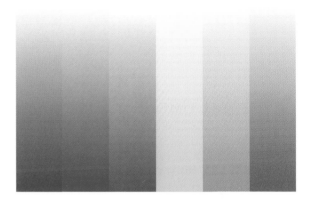

9

Yellow Zone

Yellows take Purples a step farther. Both still sit between easy and hard in intensity, with ratings of perceived exertion (RPE) in the 5 to 7 range. But Yellow workouts are longer, lasting more than 30 minutes or typically 4-plus miles.

We introduce no new elements to your program in this chapter, so you already know the types of workouts here. Only their length increases, sometimes taking impressive leaps.

The 10 Yellow workouts are best suited for runners training to race at distances longer than 5 kilometers and up to a marathon. But the lower distances in this zone remain accessible to runners who aren't primarily concerned with racing, only with testing themselves against their own standards.

WORKOUT 1

1 STEADY RUN

TOTAL TIME: 50 minutes to 1 hour, 10 minutes

WARM-UP: Run an easy mile or so before starting main workout, or make workout's first mile slow.

WORKOUT

Distance: 5 miles
Time: 30-50 minutes
Pace: 6-10 minutes per mile
Effort: RPE 5
% max HR: 75-79

COOL-DOWN: Walk a few minutes, then run an easy mile or so, walk again, and stretch.

CALORIES BURNED: 500-700

COMMENTS

This should not be a time trial. The idea isn't to see how fast you can go, but only to maintain medium intensity.

STEADY RUN

TOTAL TIME: 55 minutes to 1 hour, 20 minutes

WARM-UP: Run an easy mile or so before starting main workout, or make the workout's first mile slow.

WORKOUT

Distance: 6 miles
Time: 36 minutes to 1 hour
Pace: 6-10 minutes per mile
Effort: RPE 5
% max HR: 75-79

COOL-DOWN: Walk a few minutes, then run an easy mile or so, walk again, and stretch.

CALORIES BURNED: 550-800

COMMENTS

Do this workout only if you can complete the 6 miles well under an hour. If it approaches that limit, treat this as a long run at a more relaxed pace.

WORKOUT 3

3

TOTAL TIME: 1 hour, 20 minutes to 1 hour, 50 minutes

WARM-UP: Incorporate into main workout by running slow first mile or so.

WORKOUT

Distance: 10 miles
Time: 1 hour, 10 minutes to 1 hour, 40 minutes
Pace: 7-10 minutes per mile
Effort: RPE 5-6
    % max HR: 75-84

COOL-DOWN: Walk about 5 minutes, then stretch.

CALORIES BURNED: 800-1,100

COMMENTS

As noted in previous long runs, walking breaks are an acceptable supplement when going this far. Take the walks if needed, but don't count them toward the total distance. For example, in this workout you might walk 2 minutes after every 2 miles but still do the full 10 miles of running.

WORKOUT 4

LONG RUN

TOTAL TIME: 1 hour, 35 minutes to 2 hours, 10 minutes

WARM-UP: Incorporate into main workout by running slow first mile or so.

WORKOUT

Distance: 12 miles

Time: 1 hour, 24 minutes to 2 hours

Pace: 7-10 minutes per mile

Effort: RPE 5-6
          % max HR: 75-84

COOL-DOWN: Walk about 5 minutes, then stretch.

CALORIES BURNED: 950-1,300

COMMENTS

Now that you're spending more than an hour and a half on the road, you might appreciate some company. Seek out a companion or group to share this time.

WORKOUT 5

LONG RUN

TOTAL TIME: 1 hour, 55 minutes to 2 hours, 40 minutes

WARM-UP: Incorporate into main workout by running slow first mile or so.

WORKOUT

Distance: 15 miles

Time: 1 hour, 45 minutes to 2 hours, 30 minutes

Pace: 7-10 minutes per mile

Effort: RPE 5-6
% max HR: 75-84

COOL-DOWN: Walk about 5 minutes, then stretch.

CALORIES BURNED: 1,150-1,600

COMMENTS

The long runs in this range are likely to be taken only by people who are training for a marathon. And you should go to these lengths only at 2- to 3-week intervals.

WORKOUT 6

LONG RUN

TOTAL TIME: 2 hours, 15 minutes to 3 hours, 10 minutes

WARM-UP: Incorporate into main workout by running slow first mile or so.

WORKOUT

Distance: 18 miles

Time: 2 hours, 6 minutes to 3 hours

Pace: 7-10 minutes per mile

Effort: RPE 5-6

% max HR: 75-84

COOL-DOWN: Walk about 5 minutes, then stretch.

CALORIES BURNED: 1,350-1,900

COMMENTS

This long run equates to the metric 30K, which is the last standard racing distance before the marathon. Take this run in a race if you can find one.

7

LONG RUN

LONG RUN

TOTAL TIME: 2 hours, 30 minutes to 3 hours, 30 minutes

WARM-UP: Incorporate into main workout by running slow first mile or so.

WORKOUT

Distance: 20 miles

Time: 2 hours, 20 minutes to 3 hours, 20 minutes

Pace: 7-10 minutes per mile

Effort: RPE 5-6
% max HR: 75-84

COOL-DOWN: Walk about 5 minutes, then stretch.

CALORIES BURNED: 1,500-2,100

COMMENTS

Some runners go even farther than this while preparing for marathons. But most make this their stopping point in training and trust the excitement of the race to carry them the final 6 miles.

FARTLEK RUN

TOTAL TIME: 55 minutes to 1 hour, 10 minutes

8

WARM-UP: Run slow mile or so before starting main workout, or make workout's first mile slow.

WORKOUT

Distance: 5 miles
Time: 35-50 minutes
Pace: Varied, averaging 7-10 minutes per mile
Effort: Average RPE 6 (2-10 range)
      % max HR: 60-100

COOL-DOWN: Walk a few minutes, then run a slow mile or so, walk again, and stretch.

CALORIES BURNED: 550-700

COMMENTS

Because of its length, this workout can be quite taxing. Therefore, don't overdo the fast segments. Spread them out more than you would in a shorter fartlek run.

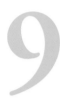

FARTLEK RUN
TOTAL TIME: 1 hour to 1 hour, 20 minutes

WARM-UP: Run a slow mile or so before starting main workout, or make workout's first mile slow.

WORKOUT

Distance: 6 miles

Time: 42 minutes to 1 hour

Pace: Varied, averaging 7-10 minutes per mile

Effort: Average RPE 6 (2-10 range)
% max HR: 60-100

COOL-DOWN: Walk a few minutes, then run a slow mile or so, walk again, and stretch.

CALORIES BURNED: 600-800

COMMENTS

A fartlek run this long is recommended only for advanced runners who are racing at distances well beyond 10 kilometers.

WORKOUT 10

UNDERDISTANCE INTERVALS
TOTAL TIME: About 1 hour

WARM-UP: Run an easy mile or 2, walk a few minutes, then take 4 to 6 100-meter strides with walk-jog 100s between, and walk again before starting main workout.

WORKOUT

Distance: Fast segments total 4-5 miles.

Recovery: Walk or jog equal distance between intervals 800 meters and shorter, and stay at 800 walk-jog for longer intervals.

Time: Fast segments total 30 minutes or more.

Pace: Date pace for your chosen distance

Effort: RPE 5-7
% max HR: 75-89

COOL-DOWN: Walk a few minutes, then run an easy mile or 2, walk again, and stretch.

CALORIES BURNED: 600-800

COMMENTS

This workout is underdistance in relation to your racing distance. A sample for a 10-kilometer runner might be 4000 meters at DP, walk-jog 800, 1500 at DP, walk-jog 800. Total distance of fast segments is 5500 meters, or about 3.3 miles.

		Summary Table		
		Yellow Zone Workouts		
Workout	**Description**	**Duration**	**Distance**	**Intensity**
1	Steady run	30-50 minutes	5 miles	RPE: 5 % max HR: 75-79
2	Steady run	36-60 minutes	6 miles	RPE: 5 % max HR: 75-79
3	Long run	70-100 minutes	10 miles	RPE: 5-6 % max HR: 75-84
4	Long run	84-120 minutes	12 miles	RPE: 5-6 % max HR: 75-84
5	Long run	105-150 minutes	15 miles	RPE: 5-6 % max HR: 75-84
6	Long run	126-180 minutes	18 miles	RPE: 5-6 % max HR: 75-84
7	Long run	140-200 minutes	20 miles	RPE: 5-6 % max HR: 75-84
8	Fartlek run	35-50 minutes	5 miles	RPE: 6 (average) % max HR: 60-100
9	Fartlek run	42-60 minutes	6 miles	RPE: 6 (average) % max HR: 60-100
10	UD intervals	30 minutes or more	4-5 miles	RPE: 5-7 % max HR: 75-89

You're now leaving the medium-intensity zone. If you passed the Purple and Yellow tests, you're ready for the most intense workouts this book has to offer.

10

Orange Zone

Oranges enter the zone of race-like intensity. In a word, this running is *hard*.

It's as hard as you're capable of running right now. But this doesn't mean it's foolhardy. You're asked to run only at the intensity you're trained to run.

This zone's ratings of perceived exertion (RPE) range from 8 to the scale's maximum of 10. The duration of these runs is 30 minutes or less, or typically 1 to 3 miles.

Many of the interval sessions look similar to those in chapter 8. But remember, their intensity level has now gone up a notch.

The 10 Orange workouts are keyed toward runners who are aiming to improve their performances at the shorter distances, those 5 kilometers and below. Included here are two new elements:

- **Date-Pace Run.** This workout is the closest you come to race effort without actually racing. It's what we sometimes refer to as a time trial.

  You run a distance of 1500 to 5000 meters at date pace. If you exceed your old DP, this time becomes the new level on which you base future training.

- **Short-Distance Race.** This is where you formally put yourself on the line in the company of other runners.

  Race a distance of 1500 to 5000 meters as fast as your training will allow. Try to improve upon your date pace and reach for your goal pace.

1

GOAL-PACE/DATE-PACE INTERVALS
TOTAL TIME: 40 minutes to 1 hour

WARM-UP: Run an easy mile or 2, walk a few minutes, then take 4 to 6 100-meter strides with walk-jog 100s between, and walk again before starting main workout.

WORKOUT

Distance: Fast segments total 1-3 miles.
Recovery: Walk or jog equal distance between intervals 800 meters and shorter, and stay at 800 walk-jog for longer intervals.
Time: Fast segments total 30 minutes or less.
Pace: Mix goal pace and date pace for your chosen distance.
Effort: RPE 8-10
         % max HR: 90-100

COOL-DOWN: Walk a few minutes, then run an easy mile or 2, walk again, and stretch.

CALORIES BURNED: 400-600

COMMENTS

Goal-pace/date-pace interval workout for a 5000-meter runner might be 4 × 600 meters at GP with 600 walk-jog between, and 4 × 600 at DP with 600 walk-jog. Total distance of fast segments is 4800 meters, or about 3 miles.

WORKOUT 2

GOAL-PACE INTERVALS
TOTAL TIME: 40 minutes to 1 hour

2

WARM-UP: Run an easy mile or 2, walk a few minutes, then take 4 to 6 100-meter strides with walk-jog 100s between, and walk again before starting main workout.

WORKOUT

Distance: Fast segments total 1-3 miles.
Recovery: Walk or jog equal distance between intervals 800 meters and shorter, and stay at 800 walk-jog for longer intervals.
Time: Fast segments total 30 minutes or less.
Pace: Goal pace for your chosen distance
Effort: RPE 8-10
%% max HR: 90-100

COOL-DOWN: Walk a few minutes, then run an easy mile or 2, walk again, and stretch.

CALORIES BURNED: 400-600

COMMENTS

Goal-pace interval workout for a mile runner might be 6 × 400 meters at GP with walk-jog 400s between. Total distance of fast segments is 2400 meters, or about 1.5 miles.

WORKOUT 3

3

UNDERDISTANCE INTERVALS
TOTAL TIME: 40 minutes to 1 hour

WARM-UP: Run an easy mile or 2, walk a few minutes, then take 4 to 6 100-meter strides with walk-jog 100s between, and walk again before starting main workout.

WORKOUT

Distance: Fast segments total 1-3 miles.
Recovery: Walk or jog equal distance between intervals 800 meters and shorter, and stay at 800 walk-jog for longer intervals.
Time: Fast segments total 30 minutes or less.
Pace: Date pace for your chosen distance
Effort: RPE 8-10
      % max HR: 90-100

COOL-DOWN: Walk a few minutes, then run an easy mile or 2, walk again, and stretch.

CALORIES BURNED: 400-600

COMMENTS

Underdistance interval workout for a 5000-meter runner might be 4000 meters at DP, walk-jog 800, 1500 at DP with walk-jog 800. Total distance of fast segments is 5500 meters, or about 3.3 miles.

WORKOUT 4

RHYTHM INTERVALS
TOTAL TIME: 40 minutes to 1 hour

4

WARM-UP: Run an easy mile or 2, walk a few minutes, then take 4 to 6 100-meter strides with walk-jog 100s between, and walk again before starting main workout.

WORKOUT

Distance: Fast segments total 1-3 miles.
Recovery: Dispense with normal walk-jogs between intervals; all at fast pace.
Time: Fast segments total 30 minutes or less.
Pace: Alternate goal pace with slightly slower than date pace.
Effort: RPE 8-10
% max HR: 90-100

COOL-DOWN: Walk a few minutes, then run an easy mile or 2, walk again, and stretch.

CALORIES BURNED: 400-600

COMMENTS

A sample workout for a mile runner might be 10 × 200, alternating between GP and slower than DP. Total distance of fast segments is 2000 meters, or about 1.2 miles.

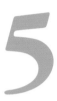

WORKOUT 5

5

DATE-PACE RUN
TOTAL TIME: 30-40 minutes

WARM-UP: Run an easy mile or 2, walk a few minutes, then take 4 to 6 100-meter strides with walk-jog 100s between, and walk again before starting main workout.

WORKOUT
Distance: 1 mile
Time: 5-10 minutes
Pace: 5-10 minutes per mile
Effort: RPE 8-10
% max HR: 90-100

COOL-DOWN: Walk a few minutes, then run an easy mile or 2, walk again, and stretch.

CALORIES BURNED: 300-400

COMMENTS
Here, you mimic the conditions of a race. The difference is that outside the formal competitive setting you feel less pressure and don't push yourself quite so hard.

WORKOUT 6

DATE-PACE RUN
TOTAL TIME: 35-50 minutes

6

WARM-UP: Run an easy mile or 2, walk a few minutes, then take 4 to 6 100-meter strides with walk-jog 100s between, and walk again before starting main workout.

WORKOUT
Distance: 3000 meters
Time: 10-20 minutes
Pace: 5-10 minutes per mile
Effort: RPE 8-10
% max HR: 90-100

COOL-DOWN: Walk a few minutes, then run an easy mile or 2, walk again, and stretch.

CALORIES BURNED: 350-500

COMMENTS

Although the standard racing distance here is 3000 meters, you'll get the same training effect by running 2 miles because it's only about a half-lap farther on the track.

WORKOUT 7

7

DATE-PACE RUN
TOTAL TIME: 40-55 minutes

WARM-UP: Run an easy mile or 2, walk a few minutes, then take 4 to 6 100-meter strides with walk-jog 100s between, and walk again before starting main workout.

WORKOUT

Distance: 5000 meters
Time: 16-30 minutes
Pace: 5-10 minutes per mile
Effort: RPE 8-10
%max HR: 90-100

COOL-DOWN: Walk a few minutes, then run an easy mile or 2, walk again, and stretch.

CALORIES BURNED: 400-550

COMMENTS

This workout's benefit is felt most at the 5K distance. But it will also help your development at distances ranging from 3K to 10K.

WORKOUT 8

SHORT-DISTANCE RACE
TOTAL TIME: 30-40 minutes

8

WARM-UP: Run an easy mile or 2, walk a few minutes, then take 4 to 6 100-meter strides with walk-jog 100s between, and walk again before starting race.

WORKOUT
Distance: 1 mile
Time: 5-10 minutes
Pace: 5-10 minutes per mile
Effort: RPE 9-10
% max HR: 95-100

COOL-DOWN: Walk a few minutes, then run an easy mile or 2, walk again, and stretch.

CALORIES BURNED: 300-400

COMMENTS

Here's where you put yourself on the line with other runners. Resist the most common mistake of racers, which is getting caught up in crowd hysteria and starting too fast. Try to make the first and last halves of the race nearly equal in time.

SHORT-DISTANCE RACE
TOTAL TIME: 35-50 minutes

WARM-UP: Run an easy mile or 2, walk a few minutes, then take 4 to 6 100-meter strides with walk-jog 100s between, and walk again before starting race.

WORKOUT

Distance: 3000 meters

Time: 10-20 minutes

Pace: 5-10 minutes per mile

Effort: RPE 9-10

       % max HR: 95-100

COOL-DOWN: Walk a few minutes, then run an easy mile or 2, walk again, and stretch.

CALORIES BURNED: 350-500

COMMENTS

The 3K most closely resembles in length the 12-minute test that you took at the start of this book. See how much your estimated VO_2 max reading has improved since that first test.

WORKOUT 10

SHORT-DISTANCE RACE
TOTAL TIME: 40-55 minutes

10

WARM-UP: Run an easy mile or 2, walk a few minutes, then take 4 to 6 100-meter strides with walk-jog 100s between, and walk again before starting race.

WORKOUT

Distance: 5000 meters
Time: 16-30 minutes
Pace: 5-10 minutes per mile
Effort: RPE 9-10
    % max HR: 95-100

COOL-DOWN: Walk a few minutes, then run an easy mile or 2, walk again, and stretch.

CALORIES BURNED: 400-500

COMMENTS

Road racing traditionally begins with the 5K distance. This race provides excellent speedwork for all the longer events.

Summary Table			
Orange Zone Workouts			
Workout **Description**	**Duration**	**Distance**	**Intensity**
1 GP/DP intervals or less	30 minutes	1-3 miles	RPE: 8-10 % max HR: 90-100
2 GP intervals	30 minutes or less	1-3 miles	RPE: 8-10 % max HR: 90-100
3 UD intervals	30 minutes or less	1-3 miles	RPE: 8-10 % max HR: 90-100
4 Rhythm intervals	30 minutes or less	1-3 miles	RPE: 8-10 % max HR: 90-100
5 Date-pace run	5-10 minutes	1 mile	RPE: 8-10 % max HR: 90-100
6 Date-pace run	10-20 minutes	3 kilometers	RPE: 8-10 % max HR: 90-100
7 Date-pace run	16-30 minutes	5 kilometers	RPE: 8-10 % max HR: 90-100
8 SD race	5-10 minutes	1 mile	RPE: 9-10 % max HR: 95-100
9 SD race	10-20 minutes	3 kilometers	RPE: 9-10 % max HR: 95-100
10 SD race	16-30 minutes	5 kilometers	RPE: 9-10 % max HR: 95-100

Those are your short-hard sessions. The longest and hardest are all that remain.

11

Red Zone

Reds represent your greatest efforts in terms of intensity and duration, and in their potential rewards. These workouts carry ratings of perceived exertion (RPE) of 8 to 10, and they last longer than 30 minutes or 4 miles.

The 10 Red sessions work best to prepare runners who race above the 5-kilometer distance. Many of the workouts actually occur as long-distance races.

These are full efforts under formal racing conditions. You try to improve your date pace or reach your goal pace at distances as long as a marathon.

WORKOUT 1

1

UNDERDISTANCE INTERVALS
TOTAL TIME: About 1 hour

WARM-UP: Run an easy mile or 2, walk a few minutes, then take 4 to 6 100-meter strides with walk-jog 100s between, and walk again before starting main workout.

WORKOUT

Distance: Fast segments total 4-5 miles.

Recovery: Walk or jog an equal distance between intervals 800 meters and shorter, and stay at 800 walk-jog for longer intervals.

Time: Fast segments total 30 minutes or more.

Pace: Date pace for your chosen distance

Effort: RPE 8-10
% max HR: 90-100

COOL-DOWN: Walk a few minutes, then run an easy mile or 2, walk again, and stretch.

CALORIES BURNED: 600-800

COMMENTS

These sessions are underdistance only for people who race 10 kilometers and longer. An underdistance interval workout for a 10K runner might be 5000 meters at DP with walk-jog 800; 2000 meters at DP with 800 walk-jog. Total distance of fast segments is 7000 meters, or about 4.3 miles.

WORKOUT 2

DATE-PACE RUN
TOTAL TIME: 50 minutes to 1 hour, 20 minutes

2

WARM-UP: Run an easy mile or so, walk a few minutes, then take 4 to 6 100-meter strides, and walk again before starting main workout; or incorporate warm-up into distance that follows by starting slowly.

WORKOUT

Distance: 10 kilometers
Time: 37 minutes to 1 hour, 2 minutes
Pace: 6-10 minutes per mile
Effort: RPE 8-10
      % max HR: 90-100

COOL-DOWN: Walk 5-10 minutes, then optional easy run of 1-2 miles (for advanced runners only), and stretch.

CALORIES BURNED: 500-800

COMMENTS

Feel free to substitute a date-pace run of 8K or 12K. The benefits will be almost the same as for a 10K.

WORKOUT 3

3

DATE-PACE RUN
TOTAL TIME: 1 hour, 10 minutes to 1 hour, 50 minutes

WARM-UP: Run an easy mile or so, walk a few minutes, then take 4 to 6 100-meter strides, and walk again before starting main workout; or incorporate warm-up into distance that follows by starting slowly.

WORKOUT

Distance: 15 kilometers
Time: 56 minutes to 1 hour, 33 minutes
Pace: 6-10 minutes per mile
Effort: RPE 8-10
        % max HR: 90-100

COOL-DOWN: Walk 5-10 minutes, then optional easy run of about a mile (for advanced runners only), and stretch.

CALORIES BURNED: 700-1,100

COMMENTS

The distance of this run might also be 10 miles. It is one of the few remaining standard racing distances to be run by miles instead of meters.

WORKOUT 4

DATE-PACE RUN
TIME: 1 hour, 30 minutes to 2 hours, 20 minutes

4

WARM-UP: Run an easy mile or so, walk a few minutes, then take 4 to 6 100-meter strides, and walk again before starting main workout; or incorporate warm-up into distance that follows by starting slowly.

WORKOUT

Distance: 20 kilometers
Time: 1 hour, 14 minutes to 2 hours, 4 minutes
Pace: 6-10 minutes per mile
Effort: RPE 8-10
     % max HR: 90-100

COOL-DOWN: Walk 5-10 minutes, then optional easy run of about a mile (for advanced runners only), and stretch.

CALORIES BURNED: 900-1,400

COMMENTS

Substitute a half-marathon if you wish. This commonly raced distance is 13.1 miles or 21.1 kilometers.

WORKOUT 5

LONG-DISTANCE RACE
TOTAL TIME: 45 minutes to 1 hour, 5 minutes

WARM-UP: Run an easy mile or so, walk a few minutes, then take 4 to 6 100-meter strides and walk again before starting main workout; or incorporate warm-up into distance that follows by starting slowly.

WORKOUT
Distance: 8 kilometers
Time: 30-50 minutes
Pace: 6-10 minutes per mile
Effort: RPE 9-10
        % max HR: 95-100

COOL-DOWN: Walk 5-10 minutes, then optional easy run of a mile or 2 (for advanced runners only), and stretch.

CALORIES BURNED: 450-650

COMMENTS
As the warm-up note suggests, runners see distances differently. How you approach this race depends on whether you're stepping up or down in distance, or whether you're running for speed or just to survive.

WORKOUT 6

LONG-DISTANCE RACE
TOTAL TIME: 55 minutes to 1 hour, 15 minutes

6

WARM-UP: Run an easy mile or so, walk a few minutes, then take 4 to 6 100-meter strides, and walk again before starting main workout; or incorporate warm-up into distance that follows by starting slowly.

WORKOUT

Distance: 10 kilometers
Time: 37 minutes to 1 hour, 2 minutes
Pace: 6-10 minutes per mile
Effort: RPE 9-10
          % max HR: 95-100

COOL-DOWN: Walk 5-10 minutes, then optional easy run of a mile or 2 (for advanced runners only), and stretch.

CALORIES BURNED: 550-750

COMMENTS

This is by far the most popular road-racing distance. Most runners know what 10K times mean, and you'll be asked regularly, What's yours?

WORKOUT 7

7

LONG-DISTANCE RACE
TOTAL TIME: 1 hour, 10 minutes to 1 hour, 50 minutes

WARM-UP: Run an easy mile or so, walk a few minutes, then take 4 to 6 100-meter strides, and walk again before starting main workout; or incorporate warm-up into distance that follows by starting slowly.

WORKOUT
Distance: 15 kilometers
Time: 56 minutes to 1 hour, 33 minutes
Pace: 6-10 minutes per mile
Effort: RPE 9-10
      % max HR: 95-100

COOL-DOWN: Walk 5-10 minutes, then optional easy run of about a mile (for advanced runners only), and stretch.

CALORIES BURNED: 700-1,100

COMMENTS

Don't be tempted to race—or even to train hard—the next week or two after this race. The formula runners often go by is to allow 1 day of recovery for each mile of racing—or about 10 days for a 15K.

WORKOUT 8

LONG-DISTANCE RACE
TOTAL TIME: 1 hour, 30 minutes to 2 hours, 20 minutes

WARM-UP: Run an easy mile or so, walk a few minutes, then take 4 to 6 100-meter strides, and walk again before starting main workout; or incorporate warm-up into distance that follows by starting slowly.

WORKOUT

Distance: 20 kilometers
Time: 1 hour, 14 minutes to 2 hours, 4 minutes
Pace: 7-10 minutes per mile
Effort: RPE 9-10
         % max HR: 95-100

COOL-DOWN: Walk 5-10 minutes, then an optional easy run of a mile or 2 (for advanced runners only), and stretch.

CALORIES BURNED: 900-1,400

COMMENTS

You're now running back-to-back 10Ks with no recovery period in between. You can estimate your 20K potential by multiplying a recent 10K performance by 2.1.

WORKOUT 9

9

LONG-DISTANCE RACE
TOTAL TIME: 2 hours, 5 minutes to 2 hours, 45 minutes

WARM-UP: Run briefly and easily (advanced runners only), or incorporate warm-up into distance that follows by starting slowly.

WORKOUT

Distance: 25 kilometers

Time: 1 hour, 39 minutes to 2 hours, 30 minutes

Pace: 7-10 minutes per mile

Effort: RPE 9-10
% max HR: 95-100

COOL-DOWN: Walk and stretch.

CALORIES BURNED: 1,250-1,650

COMMENTS

Races in the 15- to 20-mile range make perfect training for a marathon. It's more pleasant to run this far with a crowd than by yourself.

WORKOUT 10

LONG-DISTANCE RACE
TOTAL TIME: 3 hours, 20 minutes to 4 hours, 35 minutes

10

WARM-UP: Run briefly and slowly (advanced runners only), or incorporate warm-up into distance that follows.

WORKOUT

Distance: Marathon (26.2 miles)

Time: 3 hours, 3 minutes to 4 hours, 22 minutes

Pace: 7-10 minutes per mile

Effort: RPE 9-10
     % max HR: 95-100

COOL-DOWN: Walk and stretch.

CALORIES BURNED: 2,000-2,750

COMMENTS

This is the Mount Everest of running. Everyone who has come to the foot of it by training into the Red zone should make the final ascent someday.

		Summary Table		
		Red Zone Workouts		
Workout	**Description**	**Duration**	**Distance**	**Intensity**
1	UD intervals	30 minutes or more	4-5 miles	RPE: 8-10 % max HR: 90-100
2	Date-pace run	37-62 minutes	10 kilometers	RPE: 8-10 % max HR: 90-100
3	Date-pace run	56-93 minutes	15 kilometers	RPE: 8-10 % max HR: 90-100
4	Date-pace run	74-124 minutes	20 kilometers	RPE: 8-10 % max HR: 90-100
5	LD race	30-50 minutes	8 kilometers	RPE: 9-10 % max HR: 95-100
6	LD race	37-62 minutes	10 kilometers	RPE: 9-10 % max HR: 95-100
7	LD race	56-93 minutes	15 kilometers	RPE: 9-10 % max HR: 95-100
8	LD race	74-124 minutes	20 kilometers	RPE: 9-10 % max HR: 95-100
9	LD race	99-150 minutes	25 kilometers	RPE: 9-10 % max HR: 95-100
10	LD race	183-262 minutes	26.2 miles	RPE: 9-10 % max HR: 95-100

So there you have it—the full list of individual workouts. In Part III, we blend them together into training schedules tailored for you.

PART III

TRAINING BY THE WORKOUT ZONES

Here comes the exciting part. You learned the ingredients in Part II, and now you can combine them into a program of workouts that will lead to the improvement you seek.

The programs here are as personal as we can make them. They're based on *your* abilities and *your* goals. We start this personalizing by identifying just what those abilities are and what your goals are for the near future. These programs are built on two cornerstones: your performance level and your choice of distance.

Performance Level

Your general approach to running will probably fit into one of the three categories that follow. Choose your training schedule from chapter 13 according to the type of running that you do:

- **Beginning/Easy running** (or jogging). Consider yourself a beginning runner if you work out primarily for exercise at relatively short distances and relaxed paces. You probably average 2 to 3 miles a day in 3 to 4 workouts per week.
- **Frequent/Moderate running**. A frequent runner trains a little longer, faster, and more often than is required for exercise. You qualify for this second type of running if you enter organized races, if you average more than 3 miles a day in training, or both. Frequent runners enter races more as a participant there to enjoy the event than as serious competitors, and usually limit their distances to 10 kilometers (about 6 miles).
- **Competitive/Intense running**. Here, the emphasis shifts to setting personal records (PRs), which is usually done in a racing setting. As a competitive runner, you require more training and more raceday effort than the frequent runner does. Your distance may extend as far as a marathon.

Choice of Event

The workout program you select depends on which distance you want to run best. In chapter 13, we offer plans centered on each of the standard race distances between the mile and the marathon.

- **One mile** (1500 meters). This training also prepares you fairly well for distances of 800 to 3000 meters, or a half-mile to 2 miles.
- **5000 Meters** (five kilometers). This training also fits the needs of runners going as short as 3000 meters and as long as 10,000 meters, or 2 to 6 miles.
- **10,000 Meters** (10 kilometers). This training also meets most of the requirements of 5K to half-marathon runners, or those going 3 to 13 miles.
- **Marathon** (26.2 miles). This training also acts as preparation for distances of a half-marathon and longer.

You aren't forever wedded to one of the performance categories or to a single distance. We expect you to move about as your fitness improves and your desire to explore this sport increases.

However, your continued good health and feeling of accomplishment demand that you choose a training schedule that matches your current abilities and ambitions. Chapter 12 tells you how to devise such a program.

12

Setting Up Your Program

Challenge is necessary for improvement, but these must be challenges that the body can handle. We call this approach CBS—challenging but safe.

For example, Mary Slaney ran into trouble when she got above a certain training load. But when I tried to restrain her, she would plead, "Dick, I'm not training hard enough."

Armed with her past training results, I could say, "Mary, last year at this time you were doing a lot of work and you ran this fast. Now you're doing more and should be able to run faster." That calmed her down, and gave her the health and confidence needed to win the 1500- and 3000-meter races at the 1983 World Championships.

Our training guidelines aren't reserved for the elite. They are equally applicable to the elderly and the very young, male or female, beginners and veterans.

Listen to Your Body

Successful training is a matter of applying and adapting to stress. Apply the right amount, and you adapt. Apply too much, and you set yourself up for poor performances, injuries, and illnesses.

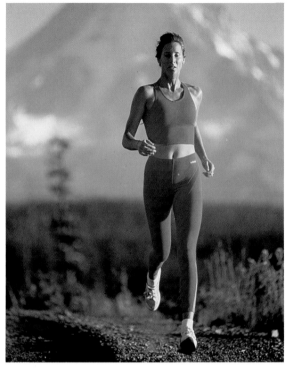

John Laptad/F-Stock, Inc.

You have to know how hard to push when.

The body will tell us what work we can and can't handle, if only we'll listen. The problem is that many active people don't know what to listen for or how to respond. By listening to what the body says and responding to its signals properly, you have a better chance of avoiding illness and injury, and maximizing performance.

The most critical signals are heart rate, body weight, and hours slept. If your heart rate is too high in the morning, you haven't recovered from the previous day's training and your body's still struggling to rebuild. If your body weight goes down too fast, you haven't rehydrated. If you don't get the sleep you need, you're going to be in trouble whether you're a world-class athlete or a recreational runner.

How can you tell if you're failing to adapt? By answering three simple questions each morning:

1. Was your resting pulse rate (taken before getting out of bed in the morning) 10% higher than normal?
2. Was your body weight (taken after voiding but before eating or drinking in the morning) 3% below normal?
3. Was last night's sleep 10% less than normal?

If you answer no to all these questions, go ahead with the challenge you've planned for yourself. If you answer yes to one question, be prepared to cut short the day's workout. If you answer yes to two questions, plan to run at an easy pace. If you answer yes to all three, take the day off. And when in doubt, be conservative!

Setting Your Goals

How fast and how far you can run is, of course, determined by how fit you are. To make that judgment, you need to take a few essential numerical readings.

$\dot{V}O_2max$

This key reading can be estimated from results of a recent 12-minute running test (see chapter 3 for instructions) or from timed runs at a number of other distances.

Table 12.1 lists running performances that correspond to various $\dot{V}O_2$ levels. The first two columns indicate laps and miles (or kilometers) run in the 12-minute test. The third column lists $\dot{V}O_2$ readings for that test result, and the remaining columns give times you could expect to run for several distances at this level of fitness.

For example, if you ran 1.5 miles in the 12-minute test (or six laps if you ran on a track), you'll find your $\dot{V}O_2max$ estimated at 38.4. You could expect to run a single mile in 7:27 and a 5K in 24:40.

Note that this table is much more detailed than the one used to assess basic fitness in chapter 3. Use Table 12.1 to create your training program.

Pace per Mile

This is the average speed of your latest timed test effort. Locate your approximate time for that full distance in Table 12.2, then find the corresponding per-mile pace in the left-hand column. For example, if you ran 5K in 24:48, your per-mile pace was 8:00.

Only a few standard distances are included here. If yours isn't one of them, simply divide the time by the distance. For example, 12 minutes divided by 1.5 miles equals 8:00 per mile.

Training Paces

You'll run short distances in the interval workouts contained in the Purple zone and onward. Table 12.3 contains times for those distances expressed as your per-mile pace. Find your mile pace in the left-hand column, then read across for equivalent times at each of the distances listed. For example, 8 minutes per mile is a pace of 2:00 for 400 meters and 4:00 for 800 meters.

Choosing Your Schedule

Read carefully here. Each workout that you select translates into physical and emotional effort on your part. How well you choose determines how well spent that effort will be.

Whether you follow the schedules we recommend in chapter 13 or design your own, you must take the following steps in setting up a program tailored to your needs:

1. **Select a date pace (DP) for any distance**. This reflects your current fitness level, so choose the performance that is most representative of your ability. It can be a 12-minute test, a time trial at another distance, or a race of any length. Locate this time in Table 12.1.

   Example: You ran a 5K in 24:48.

2. **Select a goal pace (GP) for the distance you selected**. This is a time you are likely to improve within the next year if your training progresses at a normal pace. In Table 12.1, pick a time three or four levels faster than where you now stand and make that your goal.

   Example for the 24:48 5K: You can expect to improve to 22:44-23:11 at this distance.

3. **Find your $\dot{V}O_2$ reading for date pace**. This figure appears on the same line of Table 12.1 as the result of your recent test run.

   Example for DP 5K of 24:48: This falls closest to a $\dot{V}O_2$max of 38.4.

4. **Find your $\dot{V}O_2$ reading for goal pace**. This figure appears three or four lines below the recent date-pace reading in Table 12.1.

   Example for GP 5K of 22:44-23:11: $\dot{V}O_2$max of 41.3-42.2.

5. **Choose your current distance**. This is the one on which you want to focus your attention in the weeks and months to come. Select from any of four distances—ranging from the mile to the marathon—for which we give training schedules in chapter 13.

   Example for a 5K runner: Your next race is a 10K.

6. **Find (in Table 12.1) your date pace for the distance chosen in step 5**. If you chose the same distance as for step 1, your date pace remains the same.

   Example of a different choice: Your current DP for the 10K is predicted at 51:18.

7. **Find your goal pace for that distance in Table 12.1**. If you chose the same distance as for step 2, your goal pace remains the same.

   Example of a different choice: Your current GP for the 10K is predicted at 47:16-48:13.

8. **Indicate your performance level**. This can be beginning running, frequent running, or competitive running. Part III's introduction defines these levels, and chapter 13 offers training plans for each of them. You can use the results of the health/fitness test from chapter 3 to help you determine where to start.

    Example: You want to run your 10K in an organized race, so you place yourself in the frequent category.

9. **Select your workout schedule**. This corresponds to the distance chosen and your performance level. Indicate the page on which the sample training schedule appears in this book.

    Example: You choose the frequent running schedule for a 10K runner in chapter 13.

10. **Calculate goal pace and date pace for the timed workouts you'll be performing at various distances.** Tables 12.2 and 12.3 will help you make those calculations.

    Example: Your DP 400-meter intervals are run at about 2:04 each. This is a pace of 8:15 per mile, or 51:18 for a 10K.

You'll see a major difference between our training program and most other published plans. Theirs usually go week by week.

We feel that a single week is too short to contain all the elements—easy, steady, and long runs; intervals and fartlek; hard runs and rest—that allow you to thrive physically in training. Just as important, a week is also too brief to provide the variety of workouts that make the schedule easy on you mentally.

So all the programs in chapter 13 follow 3-week cycles. In that period, you can experience training options by the dozen.

But if you choose to deviate from our recipes and design a weekly plan, we suggest that you still follow several guidelines that support our program:

- Let your performance level determine how much, how often, and how hard you run. If you follow the beginning running programs, you'll train 3 to 4 days a week, average less than 3 miles per workout, and run harder only once each week. As a frequent runner, you'll train up to 5 days a week, average 3 to 6 miles a day, and run harder once each week. Competitive runners need to train up to 6 days a week and try one or two harder runs weekly.

- Let your ability and ambition determine how fast you run. Use the date-pace and goal-pace concepts outlined in this chapter to regulate the pace of your timed workouts.

- Let yourself have one or more easy days after each harder one
  (perceived exertion of 5 or more). Whenever you run faster than
  normal, longer than normal, or both, schedule a period of rest or easy
  running (perceived exertion of 4 or less) immediately afterward.
  Don't ever run hard 2 days in a row. Recovery is the key to making
  the harder effort work for you.

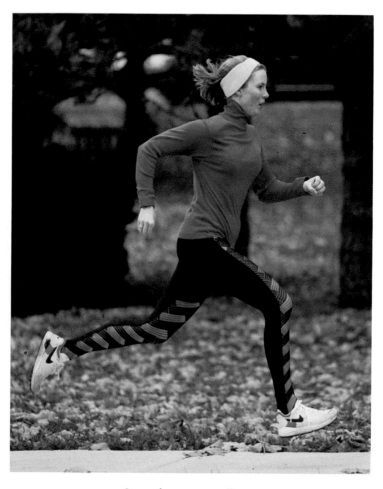

Some days you go all out.

Table 12.1
Assessing Your Abilities

Laps	Miles	(Km)	V̇O₂	Mile	5K	10K	Marathon
4	1.00	(1.60)	23.7	11:17	37:22	1:17:41	5:53:34
4-1/8	1.03	(1.65)	24.6	10:56	36:12	1:15:17	5:42:37
4-1/4	1.06	(1.70)	25.4	10:36	35:07	1:13:01	5:32:18
4-3/8	1.09	(1.75)	26.3	10:18	34:05	1:10:53	5:22:36
4-1/2	1.13	(1.80)	27.2	10:00	33:07	1:08:52	5:13:26
4-5/8	1.16	(1.85)	28.1	9:44	32:12	1:06:58	5:04:46
4-3/4	1.19	(1.90)	29.1	9:28	31:20	1:05:09	4:56:34
4-7/8	1.22	(1.95)	30.0	9:13	30:31	1:03:27	4:48:47
5	1.25	(2.00)	30.9	8:59	29:44	1:01:50	4:41:24
5-1/8	1.28	(2.05)	31.8	8:45	29:00	1:00:17	4:34:23
5-1/4	1.31	(2.10)	32.7	8:33	28:17	58:49	4:27:42
5-3/8	1.34	(2.15)	33.7	8:20	27:37	57:25	4:21:19
5-1/2	1.38	(2.20)	34.6	8:09	26:58	56:05	4:15:15
5-5/8	1.41	(2.25)	35.5	7:58	26:22	54:48	4:09:27
5-3/4	1.44	(2.30)	36.5	7:47	25:46	53:35	4:03:54
5-7/8	1.47	(2.35)	37.4	7:37	25:13	52:25	3:58:35
6	1.50	(2.40)	38.4	7:27	24:40	51:18	3:53:30
6-1/8	1.53	(2.45)	39.3	7:18	24:10	50:14	3:48:38
6-1/4	1.56	(2.50)	40.3	7:09	23:40	49:12	3:43:57
6-3/8	1.59	(2.55)	41.3	7:00	23:11	48:13	3:39:28
6-1/2	1.63	(2.60)	42.2	6:52	22:44	47:16	3:35:09
6-5/8	1.66	(2.65)	43.2	6:44	22:18	46:21	3:30:59
6-3/4	1.69	(2.70)	44.2	6:36	21:52	45:29	3:27:00
6-7/8	1.72	(2.75)	45.1	6:29	21:28	44:38	3:23:09

(continued)

Table 12.1 *(continued)*

Laps	Miles	(Km)	$\dot{V}O_2$	Mile	5K	10K	Marathon
7	1.75	(2.80)	46.1	6:22	21:04	43:49	3:19:26
7-1/8	1.78	(2.85)	47.1	6:15	20:42	43:02	3:15:51
7-1/4	1.81	(2.90)	48.1	6:08	20:20	42:16	3:12:24
7-3/8	1.84	(2.95)	49.1	6:02	19:59	41:32	3:09:04
7-1/2	1.88	(3.00)	50.1	5:56	19:38	40:50	3:05:50
7-5/8	1.91	(3.05)	51.1	5:50	19:19	40:09	3:02:43
7-3/4	1.94	(3.10)	52.1	5:44	18:59	39:29	2:59:42
7-7/8	1.97	(3.15)	53.1	5:39	18:41	38:51	2:56:47
8	2.00	(3.20)	54.1	5:33	18:23	38:13	2:53:58
8-1/8	2.03	(3.25)	55.1	5:28	18:06	37:37	2:51:13
8-1/4	2.06	(3.30)	56.1	5:23	17:49	37:02	2:48:34
8-3/8	2.09	(3.35)	57.1	5:18	17:32	36:28	2:46:00
8-1/2	2.13	(3.40)	58.1	5:13	17:17	35:55	2:43:30
8-5/8	2.16	(3.45)	59.2	5:08	17:01	35:23	2:41:04
8-3/4	2.19	(3.50)	60.2	5:04	16:46	34:52	2:38:43
8-7/8	2.22	(3.55)	61.2	5:00	16:32	34:22	2:36:26
9	2.25	(3.60)	62.2	4:55	16:18	33:53	2:34:13
9-1/8	2.28	(3.65)	63.3	4:51	16:04	33:24	2:32:03
9-1/4	2.31	(3.70)	64.3	4:47	15:51	32:57	2:29:57
9-3/8	2.34	(3.75)	65.3	4:43	15:38	32:30	2:27:54
9-1/2	2.38	(3.80)	66.4	4:39	15:25	32:03	2:25:55
9-5/8	2.41	(3.85)	67.4	4:36	15:13	31:38	2:23:58
9-3/4	2.44	(3.90)	68.5	4:32	15:01	31:13	2:22:05
9-7/8	2.47	(3.95)	69.5	4:29	14:49	30:49	2:20:15

Table 12.1

Laps	Miles	(Km)	$\dot{V}O_2$	Mile	5K	10K	Marathon
10	2.50	(4.00)	70.6	4:25	14:38	30:25	2:18:27
10-1/8	2.53	(4.05)	71.6	4:22	14:27	30:02	2:16:42
10-1/4	2.56	(4.10)	72.7	4:18	14:16	29:40	2:15:00
10-3/8	2.59	(4.15)	73.7	4:15	14:05	29:18	2:13:20
10-1/2	2.63	(4.20)	74.8	4:12	13:55	28:56	2:11:42

Mile	5K	10K	Marathon
4:00			
4:10	12:56		
4:20	13:27		
4:30	13:58	27:56	
4:40	14:29	28:58	
4:50	15:00	30:00	2:07:44
5:00	15:30	31:00	2:11:06
5:10	16:01	32:02	2:15:28
5:20	16:32	33:04	2:19:50
5:30	17:03	34:06	2:24:12
5:40	17:34	35:08	2:28:34
5:50	18:05	36:10	2:32:56
6:00	18:36	37:12	2:37:19
6:10	19:07	38:14	2:41:41
6:20	19:38	39:16	2:46:03
6:30	20:09	40:18	2:50:25
6:40	20:40	41:20	2:54:47
6:50	21:11	42:22	2:59:09
7:00	21:42	43:24	3:03:33
7:10	22:13	44:26	3:07:55
7:20	22:44	45:28	3:12:17
7:30	23:15	46:30	3:16:39
7:40	23:46	47:32	3:21:01
7:50	24:17	48:34	3:25:23
8:00	24:48	49:36	3:29:45
8:10	25:19	50:38	3:34:07
8:20	25:50	51:40	3:38:29
8:30	26:21	52:42	3:42:51
8:40	26:52	53:44	3:47:13
8:50	27:23	54:46	3:51:35
9:00	27:54	55:48	3:56:00
9:10	28:25	56:50	4:00:22
9:20	28:56	57:52	4:04:44
9:30	29:27	58:54	4:09:06
9:40	29:58	59:56	4:13:28
9:50	30:29	1:00:58	4:17:50

Table 12.2
Finding Your Per-Mile Pace

Table 12.2			
Mile	**5K**	**10K**	**Marathon**
10:00	31:00	1:02:00	4:22:00
10:10	31:31	1:03:02	4:26:22
10:20	32:02	1:04:04	4:30:44
10:30	32:33	1:05:06	4:35:06
10:40	33:04	1:06:08	4:39:28
10:50	33:35	1:07:10	4:44:50
11:00	34:06	1:08:12	4:48:12
11:10	34:37	1:09:14	4:52:36
11:20	35:08	1:10:16	4:56:58
11:30	35:39	1:11:18	5:01:20
11:40	36:10	1:12:20	5:04:42
11:50	36:41	1:13:22	5:09:04

Table 12.3
Figuring Your Training Pace

Mile	100 M	200 M	400 M	600 M	800 M	1,000 M	1,200 M
4:00	:15	:30	1:00	1:30	2:00	2:29	2:59
4:10	:15	:31	1:02	1:33	2:05	2:35	3:06
4:20	:16	:32	1:05	1:36	2:10	2:42	3:14
4:30	:16	:33	1:07	1:40	2:15	2:48	3:21
4:40	:17	:35	1:10	1:44	2:20	2:54	3:29
4:50	:18	:36	1:12	1:48	2:25	3:00	3:36
5:00	:18	:37	1:15	1:52	2:30	3:06	3:44
5:10	:19	:38	1:17	1:56	2:35	3:13	3:51
5:20	:20	:40	1:20	2:00	2:40	3:19	3:59
5:30	:20	:41	1:22	2:03	2:45	3:25	4:06
5:40	:21	:42	1:25	2:06	2:50	3:31	4:14
5:50	:21	:43	1:27	2:10	2:55	3:38	4:21
6:00	:22	:45	1:30	2:14	3:00	3:44	4:29
6:10	:23	:46	1:32	2:18	3:05	3:50	4:36
6:20	:23	:47	1:35	2:21	3:10	3:56	4:44
6:30	:24	:48	1:37	2:24	3:15	4:02	4:51
6:40	:25	:50	1:40	2:28	3:20	4:09	4:59
6:50	:26	:51	1:42	2:32	3:25	4:15	5:06

Table 12.3

Mile	100 M	200 M	400 M	600 M	800 M	1,000 M	1,200 M
7:00	:26	:52	1:45	2:36	3:30	4:21	5:14
7:10	:26	:53	1:47	2:40	3:35	4:27	5:21
7:20	:27	:55	1:50	2:44	3:40	4:33	5:29
7:30	:28	:56	1:52	2:48	3:45	4:40	5:36
7:40	:28	:57	1:55	2:52	3:50	4:46	5:44
7:50	:29	:58	1:57	2:56	3:55	4:52	5:51
8:00	:30	1:00	2:00	3:00	4:00	4:58	5:59
8:10	:30	1:01	2:02	3:04	4:05	5:05	6:06
8:20	:31	1:02	2:05	3:08	4:10	5:11	6:14
8:30	:31	1:03	2:07	3:12	4:15	5:17	6:21
8:40	:32	1:05	2:10	3:15	4:20	5:23	6:29
8:50	:33	1:06	2:12	3:18	4:25	5:29	6:36
9:00	:33	1:07	2:15	3:22	4:30	5:36	6:44
9:10	:34	1:08	2:17	3:26	4:35	5:42	6:51
9:20	:35	1:10	2:20	3:30	4:40	5:48	6:59
9:30	:35	1:11	2:22	3:33	4:45	5:54	7:06
9:40	:36	1:12	2:25	3:36	4:50	6:00	7:14
9:50	:36	1:13	2:27	3:40	4:55	6:07	7:21

(continued)

Table 12.3 (continued)

Mile	100 M	200 M	400 M	600 M	800 M	1,000 M	1,200 M
10:00	:37	1:15	2:30	3:45	5:00	6:12	7:30
10:10	:38	1:16	2:32	3:49	5:05	6:18	7:37
10:20	:39	1:18	2:35	3:53	5:10	6:24	7:45
10:30	:39	1:19	2:37	3:56	5:15	6:30	7:52
10:40	:40	1:20	2:40	4:00	5:20	6:36	8:00
10:50	:40	1:21	2:42	4:03	5:25	6:42	8:07
11:00	:41	1:23	2:45	4:07	5:30	6:49	8:15
11:10	:42	1:24	2:47	4:11	5:35	6:55	8:22
11:20	:42	1:25	2:50	4:15	5:40	7:01	8:30
11:30	:43	1:26	2:52	4:18	5:45	7:07	8:37
11:40	:44	1:28	2:55	4:23	5:50	7:13	8:45
11:50	:45	1:29	2:57	4:26	5:55	7:20	8:52

13

Sample Running Programs

One training schedule doesn't fit everyone, so we're offering many choices here. Nine different schedules span the three levels of performance.

Each schedule is keyed to improving your running at a specific distance from 1 mile on up. We have a plan for you whether you approach this sport is as a beginning runner, a frequent runner, or a competitive runner.

Beginning Running Programs

Beginning running also goes by the name *jogging*, a term that some runners find distasteful. The difference between jogging and running is more an attitude than a pace.

As a beginning runner or jogger, you probably work out purely for the aerobic benefits, weight control, stress management, and similar personal-fitness reasons. You ignore the competitive side of the sport.

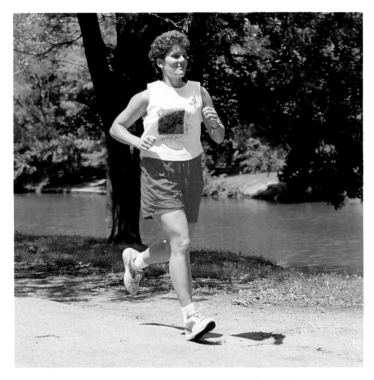

A beginning runner, out to sample the benefits of the sport.

The schedules in this chapter aim to improve your performances in the mile and 5000 meters. They offer an average of about four workouts a week at 3 miles or less per workout, with less than one of the workouts being a hard run. Hard means that it reaches into the Orange zone (high intensity, short duration). The remaining runs fall into the low-intensity Green and Blue, and medium-intensity Purple and Yellow zones.

A note for runners new to the sport: You aren't expected to enter these programs unprepared. Make sure you build up gradually to 3 easy, continuous miles before launching a schedule like ours.

One-Mile Schedule

This 3-week cycle of training is keyed to your actual or predicted mile or 1500-meter time, as determined in chapter 12. The schedule will also prepare you for other distances in the 800- to 3000-meter range.

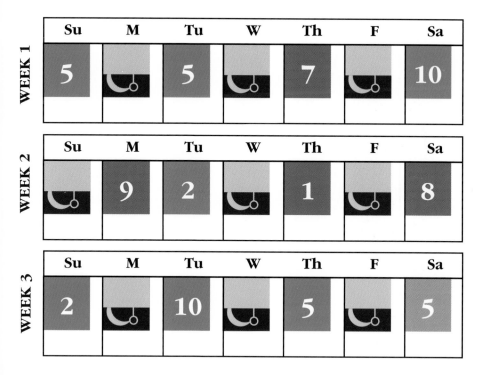

5000-Meter Schedule

This 3-week cycle of training is keyed to your actual or predicted 5-kilometer time, as determined in chapter 12. The schedule will also prepare you for other distances in the 3000- to 10,000-meter range.

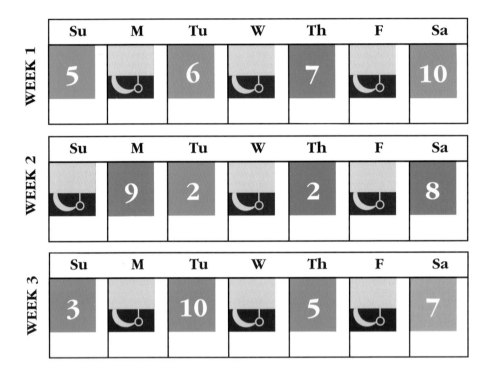

Frequent Running Programs

Frequent running takes the next step beyond simply exercising. This runner goes a little farther and runs more often than is recommended for beginning running. In other words, frequent runners find excitement in doing more than minimum amounts. They start to explore more of the sport's possibilities.

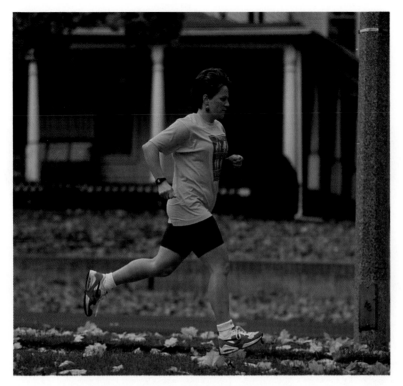

A frequent runner, testing herself more and more.

You may move into the racing arena. Frequent runners make up most of the field at any road race, and they are there more for the company of other runners than to compete. Don't let the term "race" scare you. The racing effort itself is similar to what you might do alone in training.

The schedules in this chapter aim to improve your performances in the mile, 5000 meters, and 10,000 meters. They offer an average of about five workouts a week at 3 to 6 miles per workout (depending on your choice of schedule), with one of the workouts being a hard run. Hard means that it reaches into the high-intensity Orange (short duration) or Red (long duration) zones. The remaining runs are divided among the other 4 zones of low and medium intensity. These schedules also offer an option on some days—choose one or the other where two workouts are separated by a slash mark, i.e. 5/8.

One-Mile Schedule

This 3-week cycle of training is keyed to your actual or predicted mile or 1500-meter time, as determined in chapter 12. The schedule will also prepare you for other distances in the 800- to 3000-meter range.

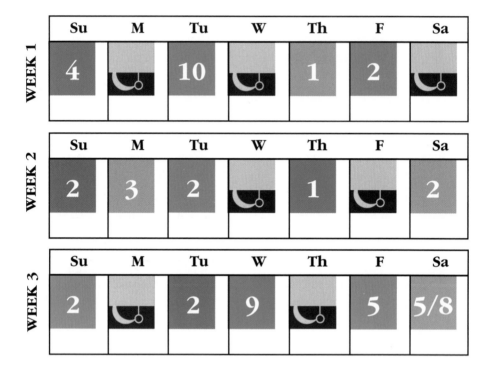

5000-Meter Schedule

This 3-week cycle of training is keyed to your actual or predicted 5-kilometer time, as determined in chapter 12. The schedule will also prepare you for other distances in the 3000- to 10,000-meter range.

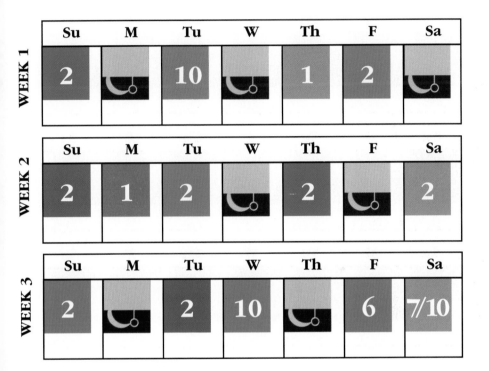

10,000-Meter Schedule

This 3-week cycle of training is keyed to your actual or predicted 10-kilometer time, as determined in chapter 12. The schedule will also prepare you for other distances in the 5000-meter to half-marathon range.

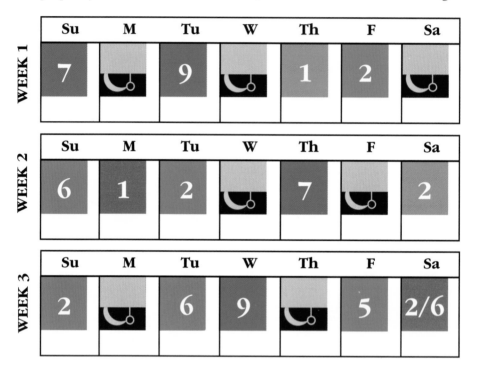

Competitive Running Programs

You're competing with yourself and your own previous performances here. You aren't required to beat anyone in head-to-head competition. Your objective is to set personal records. Doing this requires some training that goes well beyond the minimum requirements for staying aerobically fit.

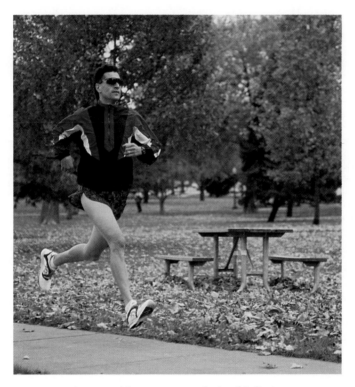

A competitive runner, exploring his limits.

The schedules in this chapter aim to improve your performances in the mile, 5000 meters, 10,000 meters, and marathon. They offer an average of about six workouts a week at 5 or more miles per workout (how much more depends on your choice of schedule), with one or two of the workouts being a hard run. Hard means that it reaches into the high-intensity Orange (short duration) or Red (long duration) zones. The remaining workouts are 4 zones of low and medium intensity.

One-Mile Schedule

This 3-week cycle of training is keyed to your actual or predicted mile or 1500-meter time, as determined in chapter 12. The schedule will also prepare you for other distances in the 800- to 3000-meter range.

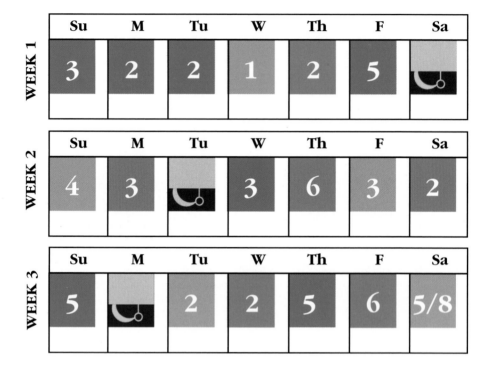

5000-Meter Schedule

This 3-week cycle of training is keyed to your actual or predicted 5-kilometer time, as determined in chapter 12. The schedule will also prepare you for other distances in the 3000- to 10,000-meter range.

	Su	M	Tu	W	Th	F	Sa
WEEK 1	6	3	3	1	2	6	⌣

	Su	M	Tu	W	Th	F	Sa
WEEK 2	4	3	⌣	6	7	1	2

	Su	M	Tu	W	Th	F	Sa
WEEK 3	6	⌣	2	2	6	6	7/10

10,000-Meter Schedule

This 3-week cycle of training is keyed to your actual or predicted 10-kilometer time, as determined in chapter 12. The schedule will also prepare you for other distances in the 5000-meter to half-marathon range.

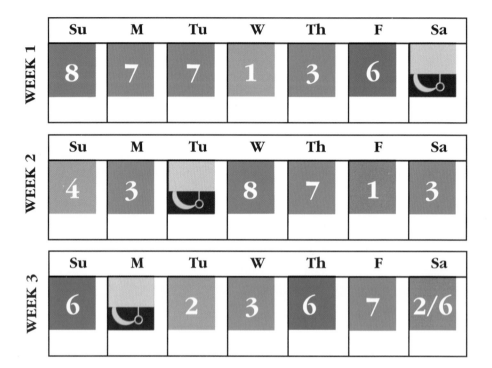

Marathon Schedule

This 3-week cycle of training is keyed to your actual or predicted marathon time, as determined in chapter 12. The schedule will also prepare you for distances of a half-marathon and longer. On several days you will complete more than one workout—these are separated with dashes, i.e. 3-4-5.

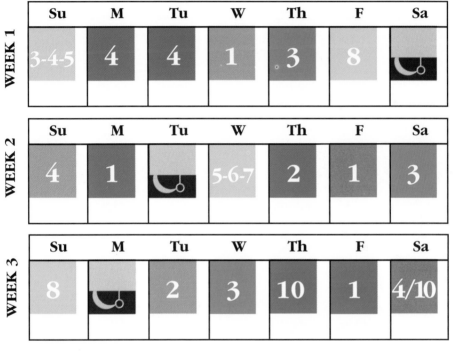

Days listed in these schedules as rest need not involve total inactivity. You want a break from the pounding of running, and any of several cross-training activities can replace a run. We'll deal with these in the next chapter.

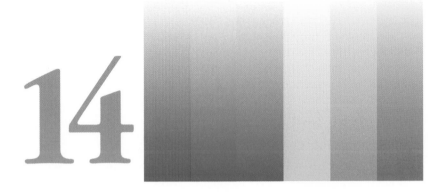

Cross-Training

Running is one of many ways to get fit. We recommend that you mix fitness activities. Overspecialization can lead to physical injury and psychological staleness, while variety can spice up your routine.

However, keep in mind that this is a *running* book and yours is a running-centered program. We could write a book on the merits of multisport activity, but we'll limit our discussion here to what cross-training offers you as a runner who prefers to spend most of your training time running.

Why Cross-Train?

A cross-training workout serves three major purposes for you, the runner:

1. It substitutes during injury periods. Most of the injuries that runners suffer will allow some type of alternative exercise that doesn't aggravate the problem.
2. It provides mental breaks during times when the running routine has gone flat. Substituting another activity for a few days or weeks can restore the appetite to run.
3. It provides rest-day activities. Runners rarely need pure rest on their days off from running, but only a break from the jarring effects of running.

In all cases, cross-training provides active recovery. To accomplish this, supplemental workouts generally will remain low in intensity and brief in duration.

We think of the cross-trainer as a runner who indulges in similar activities such as swimming, bicycling, and walking. Two adjuncts to the runner's program don't quite fit our definition but nonetheless are too valuable not to mention in this context.

Stretching and Strengthening

Running tends to be a tightening activity. You need to develop your flexibility in other ways, such as using the stretching program that we outlined in chapter 5.

Running also develops certain muscle groups while ignoring others. The lower body becomes quite strong, while the upper body goes relatively unexercised.

Another complication is that the one-directional action of running builds some leg muscles to a greater degree than others. Strength imbalances can occur, and these can lead to injuries.

In the name of maintaining or restoring muscle balance, we highly recommend that you add strength exercises to your program. These can be as simple as push-ups and sit-ups mixed into your stretching routine, or as complex as a formal weight-training workout.

Other than stretching and strengthening, our only concern here is with activities that mimic the aerobic nature of running. This is your true cross-training.

Additions and Substitutions

We're assuming that running is your first choice as a fitness activity. But we also know that there are times when you can't run or when running itself isn't enough. What then? You select an alternative or supplemental activity.

Your choices are almost limitless. We highlight five that are most comparable to running and most accessible to runners.

Aerobics (Floor or Water)

This is a favorite of people who like company when they exercise, because this is largely an organized group activity.

Aerobics trains more muscle groups than running does, but beware of the high-impact exercises. They could hurt you, or at least not give the relief from running's pounding that you want in cross-training. Opt for low-impact (on the floor) or no-impact (in the water) aerobics routines.

Bicycling (Street or Stationary)

Runners like the street or mountain bike for many of the same reasons they like to run. It takes them outdoors on the same routes they would travel as runners and lets them explore twice as much territory as they could while running.

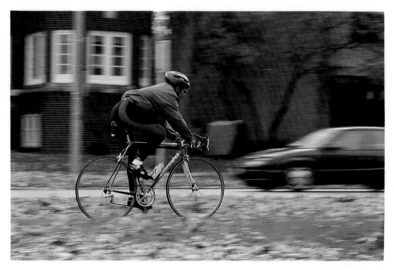

When you can't run, consider traveling even faster—on a bike.

Stationary biking lacks these pluses, of course, but provides the same great non-pounding workout. And it has the one great advantage over street biking (and street running, for that matter) of removing the threat of traffic or the rider's own carelessness.

Swimming

Unlike water running, you use the standard strokes here, preferably the crawl. The advantages of swimming over running (besides the obvious one of no impact) are that it exercises more of the body and at the same time promotes flexibility.

The disadvantage of swimming: Some runners, accustomed to looking around and talking with friends as they run, think of pool workouts as sensory deprivation.

Walking

This is the most available and least appreciated alternative. You can walk anywhere, anytime, and with very little risk of developing impact ailments. Walking delivers only about one-third the pounding of running.

However, because walking is such an efficient exercise, workouts tend to be low-intensity. The benefits are slower to come than they are with running and other cross-training activities, and you must walk longer to achieve them.

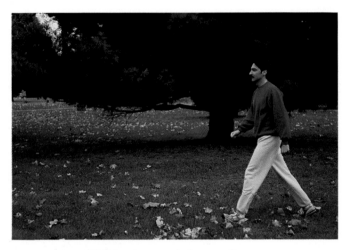

Walking is a good change of pace.

How Much Should You Cross-Train?

We recommend limiting most of the recovery-type cross-training sessions to a half-hour so you won't drain away energy from the next day's run. A half-hour's swim or bike ride is about equal in effort to a half-hour's run—provided the intensity levels are about the same.

The exception to this equal-time rule is walking. It will always be less intense than running and the other cross-training workouts. So you must walk up to twice as long (or up to an hour on recovery days) to expend a similar amount of energy.

Keep that amount small. Heed the advice of sports medicine pioneer Dr. Stan James:

"My definition of a recovery day is not doing anything that might foul up the quality running day that follows. That quality day should be a delightful, challenging, satisfying workout when you feel fresh going into it."

At best, your cross-training is refreshing physically and emotionally.

Charting
Your Progress

You're in luck. Whatever your goal is in running, you have precise ways to measure your progress toward it.

Running is imminently measurable. You work with the objective standards of distance and time, not with subjective systems of points scored or comparisons with an opponent.

Say your goal is to increase the distance of your longest run or your total weekly mileage. You know if you've done it as soon as you add laps on the track or extend a course on the street.

Or say your goal is to run a certain distance faster than ever before or to improve your overall pace. You know you've succeeded as soon as you look at your wrist-stopwatch and make quick mental calculations.

Or your goals might be even more personal. They might be centered less on how much and how fast you run than on how the running makes you look and feel.

You might run primarily to control your weight. You know if it's working each time you step on the bathroom scale.

You might run to keep your cardiovascular system in shape to supply energy and endurance throughout the day. You can tell how effectively you're training this system by checking your resting pulse rate for the stronger, slower beats you're seeking.

Changes in performance results and physical signals do occur. They come to almost everyone who seeks them, at almost any age and initial state of fitness.

But these changes don't come instantly—not overnight, not visibly in a week, and not even dramatically in a month. These are long-term reactions as the body slowly adapts to the work asked of it.

A season from now, a year from now, a decade from now . . . then you can look back proudly at how far you've progressed. But where do you look? In the records you keep. We recommend that you keep a diary, journal, or log of your workouts. That way, you capture two of running's beauties: its measurability and comparability.

Distance, time, weight, and pulse are all quickly and easily measured. By writing them down today, you'll be able to compare them accurately with what you achieve in the near and distant future. Then you'll know exactly how far you have traveled.

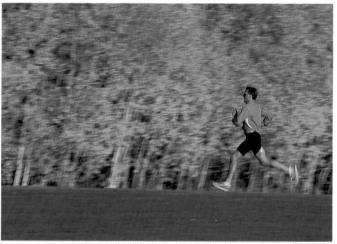

Keep thorough records of your harder runs for comparison.

Your personal accounting can be as simple as a notation on a calendar or a sheet of notebook paper. Or it can be as sophisticated as one of the published diaries or computer disks available commercially for this purpose.

You might jot down a few quick numbers. Or you may add words of commentary about the experience. Where and how you keep your records doesn't matter. Just make sure to keep them somehow and to cover the essentials.

Performance Results

Note at the very least the distance of each run and the time spent running it. Other factors you might include are the type of workout (easy, steady, fartlek, and so on), the pace per mile, the weather and terrain conditions, and how you felt.

Pay special attention to the harder workouts that may occur anywhere from every 2 or 3 weeks (for beginning runners) to twice weekly (for competitive runners). These are the timed intervals, date-pace runs, and races that give the best indications of your performance status. Compare them with previous workouts of the same type.

Physical Readings

Listen to your body. It's telling you how your training is going. Get in the habit of recording your resting pulse as you wake up each morning. A lowering of that reading over time means that your cardiovascular fitness

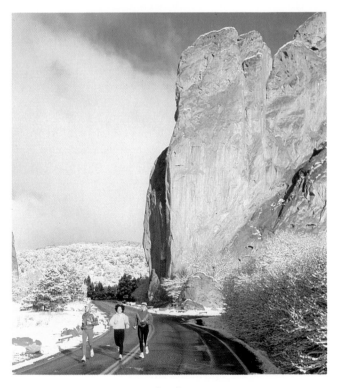

Rewards of running.

is improving. Yet a sudden jump of 5 beats or more in that heart rate can mean that you're overtrained and need a rest. Know what your norm is so you can act when it appears abnormal.

Also record your weight each morning. Most runners seek some long-term weight loss, or at least to hold their weight at its present level. But a sudden drop of three pounds or more isn't a good sign. It may again mean you've exceeded optimum training and require a break.

To get you tuned in to both schedule-planning and record-keeping, we provide a sample of a log page (see pg. 165). Write down the color and number of your planned workouts. Then, as you complete them, fill out the remaining columns. You can use the "Comments" column to record weather and terrain conditions and how you felt.

Despite the ease of putting numbers to running results, the greatest value of running can't be measured in numbers. This value is the good feeling you develop from and for running.

It's the feeling of energy and enthusiasm. It's the satisfaction of putting in solid efforts and the relaxation afterward. It's wanting to and being able to keep going and to keep coming back for more.

If running is to do all of this for you, it has to last. It's an endurance activity, to be sure, but its benefits have a short lifespan. Stop for as little as a few weeks and they vanish, but keep running and they're constantly renewed.

So your main goal is to continue. We want you to be out there running and profiting from it and enjoying it for a lifetime.

This is winning in the truest sense. You win by lasting—and by outlasting the people who injure themselves or lose interest and drop out early. As the coaches like to say, Winners never quit.

Date	Pulse / Weight		Workout zone and #	Distance	Time	Comments
S						
M						
T						
W						
Th						
F						
S						

Summary _____

_____

_____

_____

Index

About the Authors

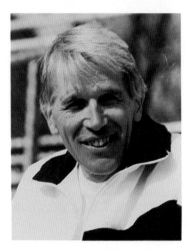

Dick Brown

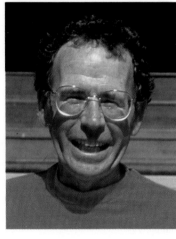

Joe Henderson

Richard L. Brown is a veteran coach and an exercise physiologist. His distinguished career began in 1963 at Bullis Preparatory School in Silver Spring, MD, where he was a three-sport coach. Brown moved to the United States Naval Academy in 1965 and spent 8 years there as an assistant professor of physical education developing personal fitness programs. From 1972 to 1978, he coached at Mt. Blue High School in Farmington, ME, and guided the school's cross-country team to two state championships and its track team to one state championship. And from 1978 to 1984 he worked for the Athletics West track and field team, first as an exercise physiologist, then as director.

In 1983, Brown was head coach of the U.S. World Championship Cross-Country Team. He also has served as a personal coach to an impressive list of world-class athletes, including Mary Decker Slaney, a National and World Champion in the 1500-meter and 3000-meter runs; Shelly Steely, a National Champion in the 3000-meter run; Debbie Lawrence, an American record holder in the racewalk at four distances; and Leslie Krichko, a member of the U.S. Olympic Cross-Country Skiing Team. Brown is one of the few coaches to have coached athletes in the Summer and Winter Olympic Games and the Paralympics.

Brown earned his PhD in exercise and movement sciences from the University of Oregon in 1992. He has received the Bruce Jenner Award for furthering the advancement of world-class track and field in the United States and the Jesse Abramson Award for Meritorious Service to Track and Field.

Joe Henderson has been writing about running for over 25 years. He is the West Coast editor and a featured columnist for *Runner's World* magazine; he was formerly senior editor for the publication. Henderson also promotes and participates in running events. He is a veteran runner with more than 700 races to his credit.

Henderson received his BA from Drake University in 1965. After graduation, he worked as an editor in the sports department at the *Des Moines Register* and later as a staff writer for *Track & Field News*. In 1967, he began his long employment with *Runner's World*. Henderson now also works as an adjunct assistant professor of journalism at the University of Oregon. He is the author of more than a dozen books on running, and he writes and produces a monthly newsletter called *Running Commentary*.

Henderson is a former executive director of the International Runners Committee, which was instrumental in placing a women's marathon in the Olympics. His honors include being inducted into the Road Runners Club of America Hall of Fame in 1978, receiving the club's journalism award in 1979, and being named a Drake University Distinguished Alumnus in 1981.

Photo Credits

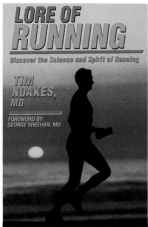
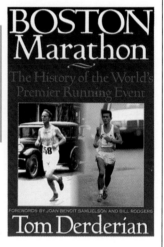
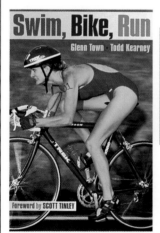